Wonders of Chinese Acupuncture

Wonders of

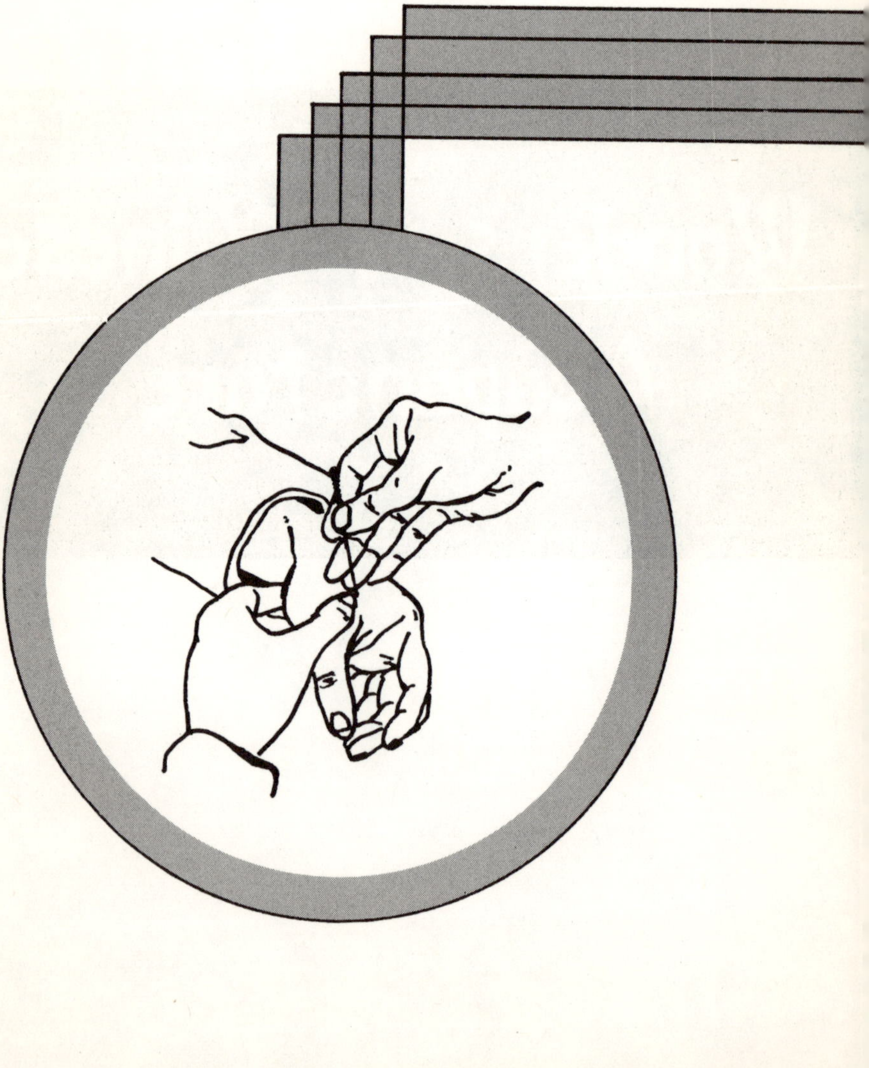

Chinese Acupuncture

by
Pedro Chan

assisted by
Albert Fields, M.D.
Samuel Pevsner, M.D.

1973
Borden Publishing Company
ALHAMBRA, CALIFORNIA

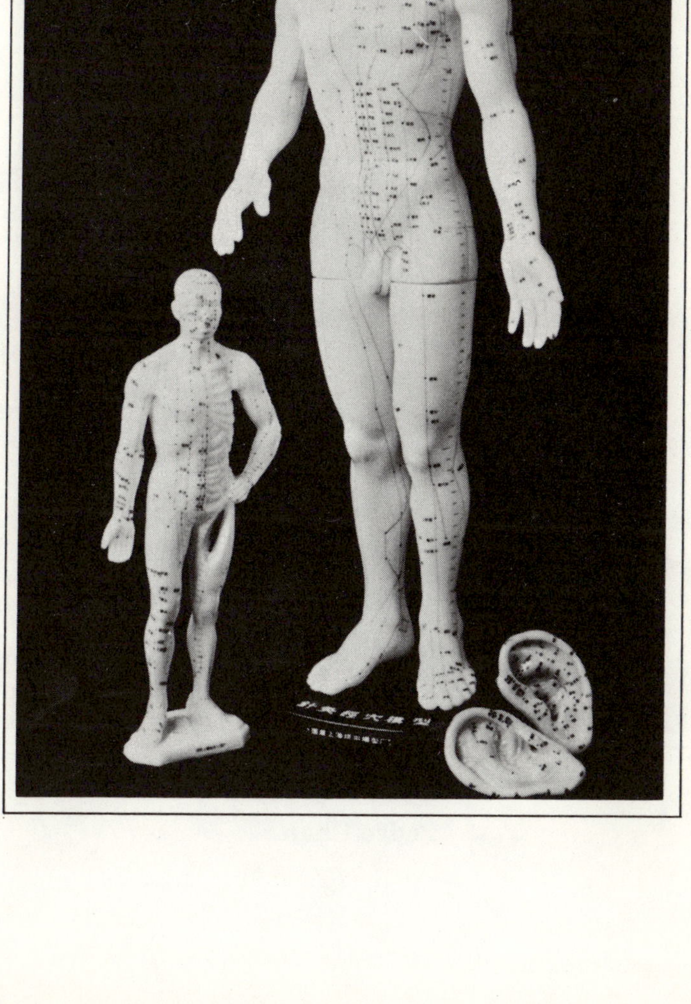

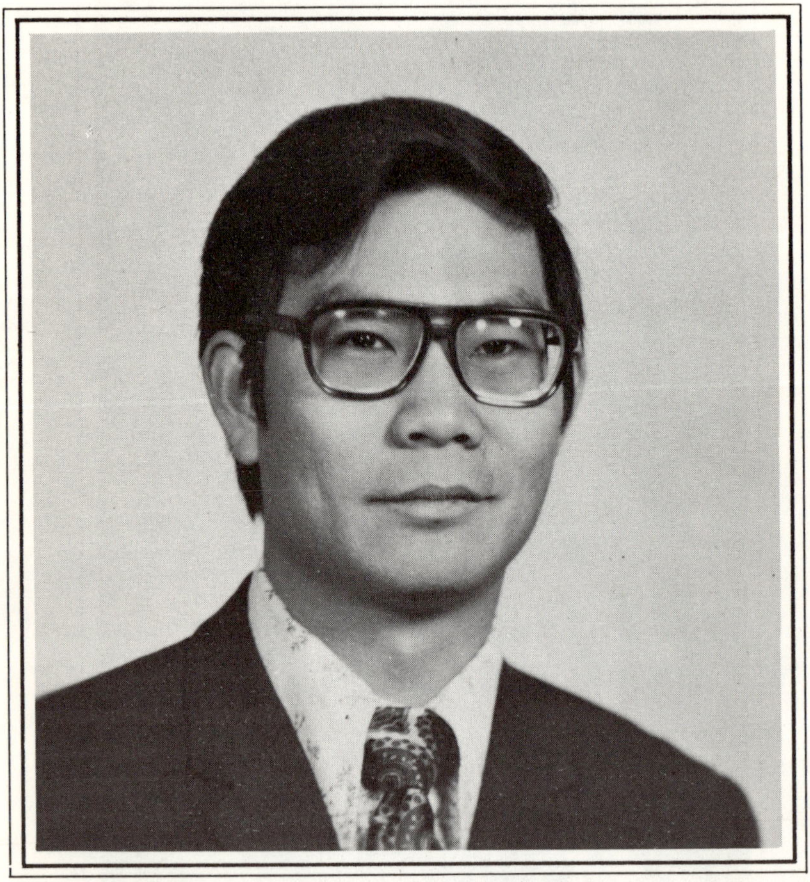

Pedro Chan

This book is dedicated to the wonderful group of people who are the future medical workers of acupuncture.

INTRODUCTION

This monograph by Pedro Chan has encompassed traditional Chinese medicine for those who desire a short but concise explanation and correlation of Chinese and Western medicine. There is no detailed explanation of the application of acupuncture in specific diseases and how their symptomatology may be altered. There is a good correlation between the two types of medical practice and the application of an integrated medical approach to patient treatment. Indeed there are many questions that need to be answered, scientific verifications to be performed and explanations and theories that need to be discussed.

Howard T. Morse, Jr., M.D.
Chairman, Department of Anesthesia,
White Memorial Medical Center

FOREWORD

"That a needle stuck into one's foot should improve the functioning of one's liver is obviously incredible. . .as a matter of empirical fact, it does happen."
A.L. Huxley 1895-1963

In 1972 Chinese needling became one of the most widely discussed topics at medical and non-medical gatherings. Mr. Pedro Chan took on the difficult assignment of explaining ancient Chinese philosophical concepts in bio-engineering terms. Mr. Chan has done a fine job in abstracting from old and new writings on acupuncture and in presenting a complicated subject in layman's language.

Since 1947 I have had published more than 20 papers on various aspects of the nine divisions of Traditional Chinese Medicine. Over 25 years ago I wrote about Acupuncture Therapy, Acupuncture Analgesia and Electro-Acupuncture!

I have found acupuncture to be effective in Caucasions as well as Orientals. In many persons, it can serve as an effective and safe anesthesia for surgical procedures. I have used it for a variety of pain syndromes. As Huxley noted, at times the insertion of needles can improve the function of a distant organ.

Acupuncture can be explained in part by counter-irritation, "distractive stimuli", trigger points "blocking", chemotaxic and physical stimuli from the inserted needle producing alterations in local and general circulation. There is indirect action on the autonomic nervous system and the endocrines through the hypothalamic-pituitary-adrenal axis.

Attention is called to the Melzack-Wall "gate control" theory, especially as modified by Wald. It is proposed that proprioceptive stimuli produced by the inserted needle are in beta fibres with thick myelin sheaths. Pain stimuli, carried in by C fibres with thin myelin sheaths, are blocked by "closing gates" in the central nervous system. Melzack and Wall originally theorized that this pain blocking occurred the synapses in the substantia gelatinosa in the dorsal horn of the spinal cord.

It is now postulated that pain impulse transmission to the cortex involves positive and negative feedback mechanisms. It is probable that in addition to a second "gate" suggested by Wald, there are "gate control" mechanisms at spino-thalamic synapses, in the medullary brain stem and in the thalamo-cortical regions.

Unlike Mr. Chan, I feel that a considerable element of suggestion and auto-hypnosis are involved in acupuncture. Arguments in support of this view cannot be discussed in detail at this time.

Our present inability to adequately explain the mechanisms of action of acupuncture does not nullify its efficacy. We should remember that aspirin often alleviates pain; except for recent glimpses provided through investigation of prostaglandins, we do not know how aspirin works. Why do pain relief and other beneficial effects of acupuncture persist after needle withdrawal? It is hoped that better answers will be provided by bio-engineers such as Mr. Pedro Chan.

"There are more things in heaven and earth, Horatio, than are dreamt in your philosophies."

W. Shakespeare 1564-1616
Hamlet, Act 1, Sc 5

Albert Fields, M.D.
Los Angeles, California

It is important for the reader to know that the subject of acupuncture is divided into two categories:

1. Acupuncture for the treatment of diseases, and
2. Acupuncture anesthesia.

It is interesting to note that acupuncture anesthesia has been used as a scientific method for only fifteen years. However, because of the dramatic nature and because it is readily demonstrable, this method of anesthesia has been unquestionably verified and documented by Western doctors.

Acupuncture for the treatment of diseases has existed for some 5000 years. However, although some of the results of treatment for diseases are also very dramatic, they have not been clearly verified and documented by Western doctors. This misunderstanding may be in part due to the reluctance of Eastern trained doctors to reveal their knowledge of acupuncture techniques and to the inability of Western trained physicians to understand and correlate the different terminology and approach that traditional Chinese medicine has both in tradition and in approach to a patient's disease and its treatment.

When the communications between Eastern and Western physicians is improved and acupuncture for the treatment of disease and for the application of anesthesia can be discussed freely, the subject may be considered similar to that of the American astronauts that had found a 5000 year old civilization and questioning whether or not the average person would be willing to accept the proposition that this civilization that had been discovered was more advanced in the field of medicine than we are today.

Samuel Pevsner, M.D.
Rio Hondo Memorial Hospital

PREFACE

Having been brought up in the traditional Chinese medical family, I have studied Chinese medicine since my early childhood. I came to the United States in 1967 and now have a B.S. in Engineering from California State University at Los Angeles.

My first booklet "Acupuncture, Electro-acupuncture, Anesthesia," was written because so many people showed a great interest in these specific topics. It can be noted that there is little material in English translation on the subject of acupuncture or on the dissertation of herbology.

An attempt to give the reader a general understanding of what acupuncture is, as well as the Chinese philosophy of traditional Chinese medicine, was presented in a book. This book was enthusiastically received, and more information and details of traditional Chinese medicine was requested. Another monograph on acupuncture and traditional Chinese medicine will more nearly meet the needs of the medical profession and laymen interested in acupuncture techniques, as a brief reference to explain the differences and conformities of both Western and traditional Chinese medicine. This book may be one of the first attempts to better explain traditional Chinese medicine and specifically that of acupuncture anesthesia in the terms of biological engineering in the United States, and explain ancient Chinese philosophy.

It is the purpose of this book to act as an introduction to Chinese medicine, providing the reader with a general idea of where acupuncture stands in the whole system of traditional Chinese medicine.

Discussion of the various aspects of acupuncture, both as a therapy and as an anesthetic technique, with the use of electro-acupuncture (even though it is still new) is included for completeness. The nervous system of Western Medicine and the meridian system of traditional Chinese medicine will be compared and the reader may make his own comparisons between the two systems. Finally, it should be understood that this addition does not intend to answer all the puzzling questions or give all the answers that the subject of acupuncture may arouse, but instead stimulate the minds of the best of both Western and traditional Chinese medicine so that a common understanding of this specific treatment of patient disease and pain may be understood.

I would like to express my deepest gratitude to Albert Fields, M.D., a Los Angeles surgeon, and Samuel Pevsner, M.D., anesthesiologist at Rio Hondo Memorial Hospital, for their great interest and critical suggestions for my book. Without their precious contributions, my work would have been impossible. I have learned a lot of biological phenomena from the class "Introduction to Bio-medical Engineering." I wish to thank my professor Leslie Cromwell, Ph.D., bio-electronic professor at California State University at Los Angeles for his continuous assistance and encouragement that enables me to apply the field of biological engineering to my knowledge of acupuncture. Sincere thanks is due individually to Kai Yan Chen, Gim Shek Ju, Wai Sang Leung, and Shui Wan Wu, acupuncture doctors, for their valuable information and kind co-operation. Also, I must not forget to thank those sweet and lovely girls who have given me a hand in preparing this manuscript; they are Allyson Chow, Susan Fung, Lena Wu, and Anna Yu.

Last of all, I am greatly indebted to Howard Morse M.D., chief anesthesiologist of White Memorial Medical Center, and president of Los Angeles County Medical Association, anesthesiology section, for all his painstaking hard work of revising my manuscript.

Pedro Chan

TABLE OF CONTENTS

LIST OF ILLUSTRATIONS

Chapter 1

Chinese Medicine

Chinese Medicine

Man needs medical care as much as he needs food, thus the history of Chinese medicine is dated back to the very beginning of the life history of the ancient Chinese people. Its whole development has covered a period of at least 5,000 years. In the ruins of ancient towns, and the remains of ancient men and articles, we can invariably find matters related to the art of Chinese medicine. From the ancient writings, and historical records, we can also relate material of immense value to medicine.

Shen Nung, the Father of Chinese Medicine, is dated back to 3,494 B.C., this is 2,000 years before Hippocrates (460-377 B.C.) Shen Nung was a sagacious emperor contributing to the field of farming as well as the study of herb-remedies. He is recognized in medical history as the first herbologist.

1.1 CHINESE PHILOSOPHY ON MEDICINE

Chinese medicine was built and enriched by a long history of practical experience, interwoven with a pattern of philosophy. Therefore, it's difficult to understand Chinese medicine without first probing into the philosophy behind it.

The Yin and Yang doctrine was first mentioned in "I Ching" (800 B.C.) and later advocated by philosophers and also applied to medical theories.

The principle of Yin and Yang is the basic principle of everything in creation. It is the root and source of life and death. Yin means the dark element, while Yang means the light element. Through their interactions and their functions, Yin and Yang are the causes of diseases which befall those who are not in harmony with these two natural forces. Only when these two natural forces within the body are in equilibrium with each other will the body remain in a healthy state. The following table shows some examples of Yin and Yang as applying to diseases:

YIN	internal	cold	void	weak
YANG	external	heat	full	strong

According to traditional Chinese philosophy, nature is divided into Yin and Yang. Also, there is a further division which puts all things into five elements: metal, water, wood, fire, and earth. It should be understood that these terms are not used by the Chinese in the actual restrictive sense, but rather as implying a corresponding idea. This is to relate oneself to its nature. There are three principal cycles. The actions and reactions among them are to bring about the ultimate balance of Yin and Yang forces. The relationship among the five elements are:

a) Creation Cycle:
Metal creates Water
Water creates Wood
Wood creates Fire
Fire creates Earth
Earth creates Metal

b) Control Cycle:
Metal controls Wood
Wood controls Earth
Earth controls Water
Water controls Fire
Fire controls Metal

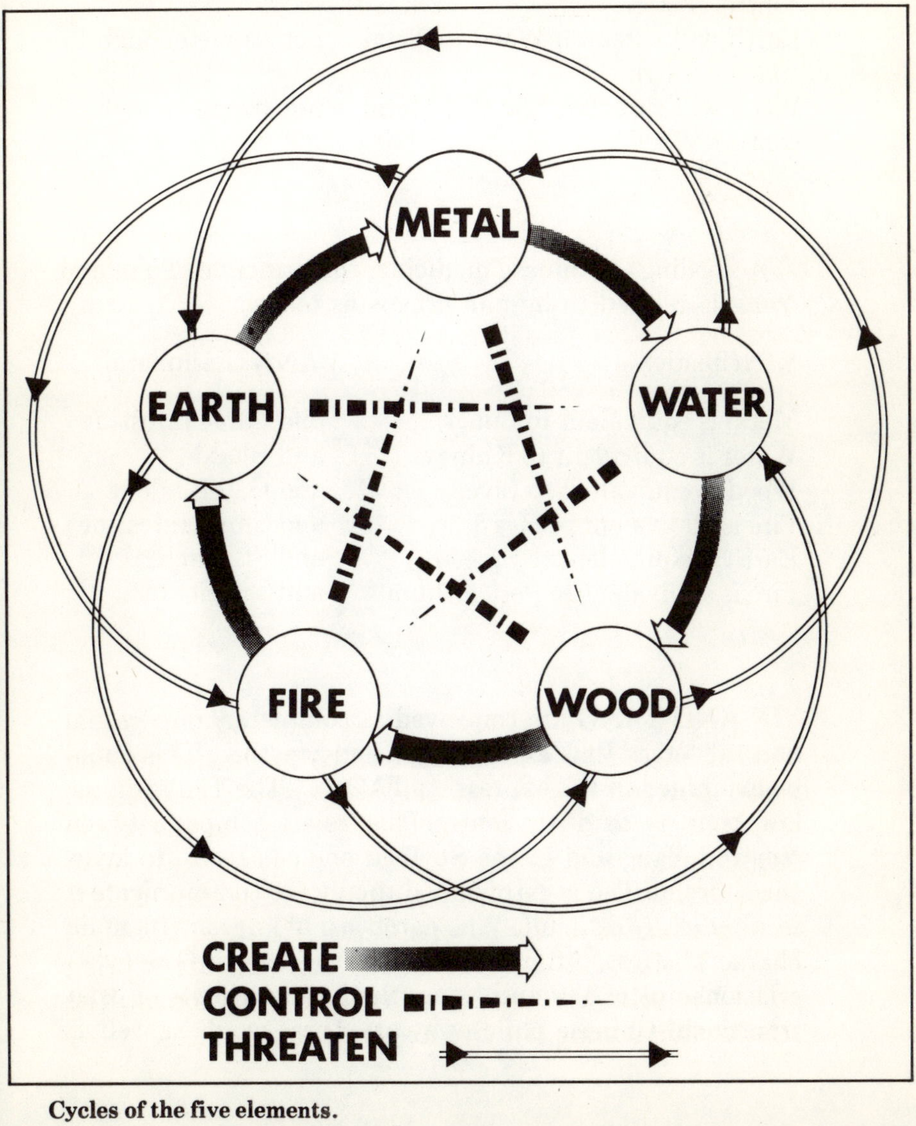

Cycles of the five elements.

c) Threatening Cycle:
Metal will threaten Fire if Fire is not strong enough to control Metal.
Fire will threaten Water if Water is not strong enough to control Fire.
Water will threaten Earth if Earth is not strong enough to control Water.
Earth will threaten Wood if Wood is not strong enough to control Earth.
Wood will threaten Metal if Metal is not strong enough to control Wood.

According to Chinese medicine, the principle of Yin and Yang is related to human organs as follows:

YIN (Inside)	**YANG** (Peripheral)
Metal is equivalent to Lungs	and Large Intestine
Water is equivalent to Kidneys	and Bladder
Wood is equivalent to Liver	and Gall Bladder
Fire is equivalent to Heart	and Small Intestine
Earth is equivalent to Spleen	and Stomach
Fire is equivalent to Pericardium	and Tri-Heater

YIN AND YANG are conceived as completely impersonal natural forces that are always found together. This could be explained in the expression TAO . . . The Tao is divine law that is said to control the relationships between Yin and Yang and in the Su Wen one can read "to know the supreme Tao is extremely difficult. To communicate it is *appallingly* difficult. Who can boast of knowing its main characteristics." After considerations of Tao and the inter-relationships of Yin and Yang, the basic concepts of what traditional Chinese philosophy are, these words as well as the inter-relationships of its component of various substances controlling one over the other in its creations cycle and control cycle are somewhat foreign, misunderstood and extremely confusing to the Western mind, however, they are not necessarily so to the traditional Chinese mind in that they are trained to think in these specific matters. It does not mean the English correlations can not be obtained for Yin and Yang and that the Tao is certainly not a substance that is completely incorrect. It is no doubt that as one continues to read traditional Chinese medicine that a concept of Western medicines certainly can be understood within the realms of traditional Chinese medicine. It is no doubt that expression of various disease processes with its recognition of diagnosis and treatment may be somewhat unusual to the Western physician, however, many of these avenues have not been extensively explored in this country as they have been in traditional Chinese medicine.

1.2 SCOPE OF CHINESE MEDICINE

Chinese medicine consists of three main categories: herbology, acupuncture and massage. Herbology uses thousands of derivatives from barks, roots, leaves, herbs, animal parts and minerals. Each item has its own curing function, but it is seldom singled out to treat the illness. Usually, a dose composed of five to ten items is the best choice. The choice of items which co-ordinates with the "natural" form of Yin and Yang, constitutes the "secret" of Chinese herbology. The herbs are then prepared as an herbal drink by boiling them in water. Western medicine has attempted in most instances to purify all drugs by specific recognization of chemical structure and pharmacological action. It is well known both in traditional Chinese medicine and Western medicine that a mixture of some drugs does have far more beneficial effects than a specific single pure drug alone. It can be suggested that in a mixture of herbal contents that are prepared in the natural form and given to patients to control their disease process may well contain drugs and combinations that are not heretofore identified.

Acupuncture has been practiced in China as long as 5000 years. It is the cure of many diseases by inserting needles into the body through specific points. One of the later techniques has advanced to surgical anesthesia or acupuncture anesthesia. A newer science involves acupuncture needles as the sole source of anesthesia in which there is applied electrical current for continued manipulation of the needle process while the patient stays awake during the operative procedures. This particular aspect of traditional Chinese medicine might be explained the Western terminology by the stimulation of intra-nuncial neurons or the administration by intru-nuncial neuron blocking drugs, causing a complete block or input of pain pattern so that there is no pain travelling up the lateral spinal thalamic or dorsal column pathways.

It should be noted that the points of acupuncture in traditional Chinese medicine are similar to those of Karate, a practice of self-defense, paralyzing or the embolization or making weaker of appointments. Comparisons of these points can well be correlated so that there is more than one aspect that can be equated as far as Western medicine is considered.

Massage is a method of treating the body by rubbing, stroking, kneading, etc. for remedial or hygienic purposes. This particular type of treatment could be considered as a less vigorous means of treating disease than acupuncture.

Beside the three main categories, there are also the methods of breathing therapy, food therapy, and mental hygiene, etc.

1.3 DIAGNOSIS IN CHINESE MEDICINE

There are four methods of diagnosing a disease in Chinese medicine. They are examinations by observation, listening, interrogation, and pulse diagnosis. Observation is based on the physical appearance of the patient including the face, eyes and tongue. Listening is based on the quality of breath and the tone of voice. The purpose of interrogation is to take into consideration the history of the patient and symptoms of the illness. Instead of giving the disease a name, the Chinese doctor attempts to determine organ and system and its dysfunction. He will study the pulses as an image from the Yin and Yang forces and determine what kind of treatment is needed to restore these two forces in balance. Once the harmonious interplay of these forces has been restored, the patient himself is able to overcome his weakness. The pulse diagnosis is both a science and an art. The diagram below depicts how pulse diagnosis is used, though in actual practice, pulse lore can only be satisfactorily learned by careful judgment and accumulated experience. Of the four diagnostic procedures, pulse examination is most important.

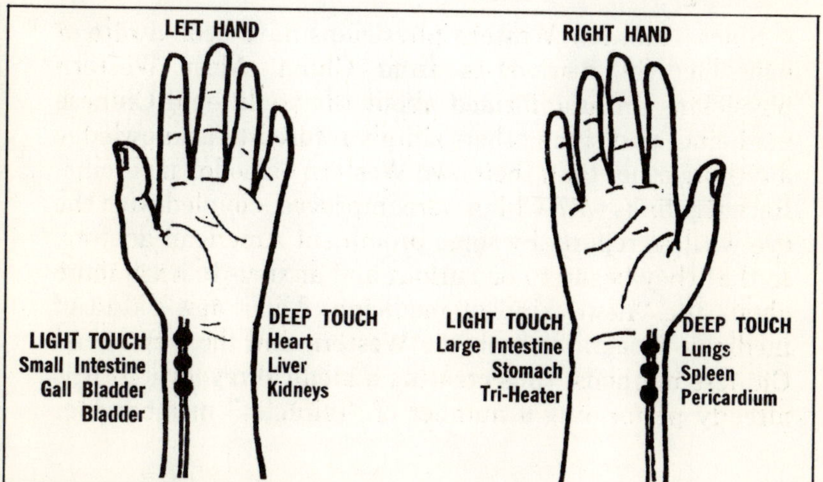

Positions of the pulses.

The above description has outlined a very general introduction to Chinese traditional medicine. It may sound rather unscientific, but it has been working for thousands of years for the Chinese people and it definitely has value. Generally speaking, it may be stated that Chinese medicine at a very early date registered important achievements in the identification, classification, and treatment of numerous disorders. Some of these discoveries were well in advance of Western medicine. Take Huai flower and ephedra for example. These two medicinal herbs that have been recorded in ancient Chinese medical treatise can benefit symptoms of high blood pressure and asthma respectively. Modern medicine has now confirmed that Huai flower contains rutin which is excellent for treating high blood pressure. Ephedra is also found that it is good for bringing immediate relief of asthma.

Sources of drugs are deemed more important than the identification of drugs so that when a source can be found a patient can be treated even if there are no medical centers in the area.

1.4 THE NEW MEDICINE IN CHINA

Since 1949, few Western physicians have been aware of new medical discoveries from China. Most Western physicians are uninformed about the traditional Chinese medicine, and some others simply refused to acknowledge anything other than their own Western orthodox medicine. Recently links with China were improved, coupled with the eye-witness reports by some prominent American doctors, so that they began to be curious and anxious to learn more about the "new" kind of medicine. This "new" kind of medicine integrates both the Western and the traditional Chinese methods, thus creating a medical revolution. It is already performing a number of "miracles" in medicine.

Let us look into the new system of combined medicine in China. It has the following features:

1. Professional Administration

It is administrators (revolutionary committee), not doctors, who lead the promotion of mutual understanding between the two schools of medicine. There can be no suspicion of favoring either the traditional or Western school. The revolutionary committee has three kinds of membership: *

(a) A representative of the People's Liberation Army.

(b) A member of the masses, which means essentially a political active and trusted worker or student.

(c) A representative of the administration or faculty.

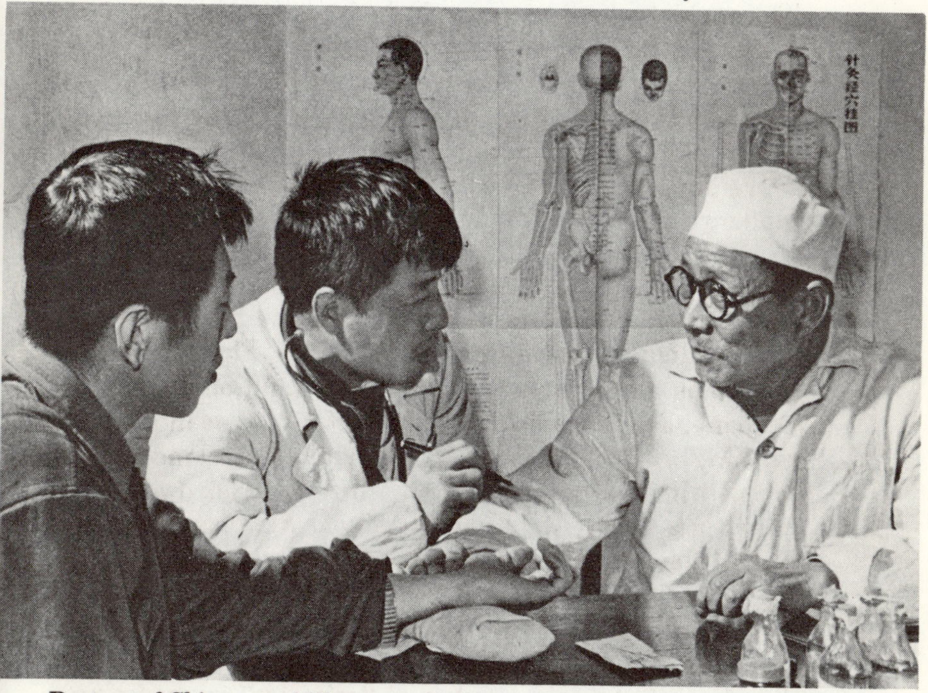

Doctors of Chinese and Western schools work hand in hand with each other. *(Medical Workers Serving the People Wholeheartedly, Foreign Language Press, Peking, 1971)*

Dimond, Grey, "Medical Education and Care in People's Republic of China," JAMA, December 6, 1971.

2. Equal Status

On one hand, the validity of traditional medicine is recognized; on the other hand, Western scientific knowledge is also respected. The traditional doctor works side by side with a colleague trained in Western medical science, each learning from the other. For example, the traditional doctor can benefit from learning to use modern diagnostic instruments. Modern scientific methods are used to analyze and compare the efficacy of the two methods, to distill the essence of each and weed out the obsolete and worthless.

3. The Period of Schooling

The period of medical schooling is shortened to about three to four years. Schooling is divided into three stages. First, while studying basic theory, the students study nursing, cleaning, and other jobs in the hospital attached to the college. This gives them a first hand knowledge of the prevention and treatment of diseases. Secondly, under guidance, they treat and prevent common diseases in rural teaching bases.* This provides training in working at the hospital. Thirdly, they return to the hospital to go into more advanced theory, improve their skill, study more seriously the complicated diseases, and to learn emergency treatment.

4. Barefoot Doctor

The barefoot doctor is a peasant who has had basic medical training and who gives treatment without leaving productive work. He has a minor dispensary at his disposal. This doctor acts as the first contact for the farmer and the connecting link to the communes' regular physicians and nurses thus providing medical service for rural people. Such doctors first appeared in the rice-growing, East China region. With their medical kits, they often went

Where they combine studies, research and clinical practice. 'Yin Chi-Wen, "Creating a New Chinese Medicine," China Reconstructs, December 1971, p. 42-44. "Health and Medical Care for the People," China Reconstructs, June 1971, p. 2 and 5.

barefoot in the fields, as was the custom. Their peasant-patients fondly called them "barefoot doctors," a term now used all over China. They also inquire for and collect medical recipes and prescriptions kept by the people as family treasures handed down from father to son. These recipes and prescriptions are then tested by scientific research.

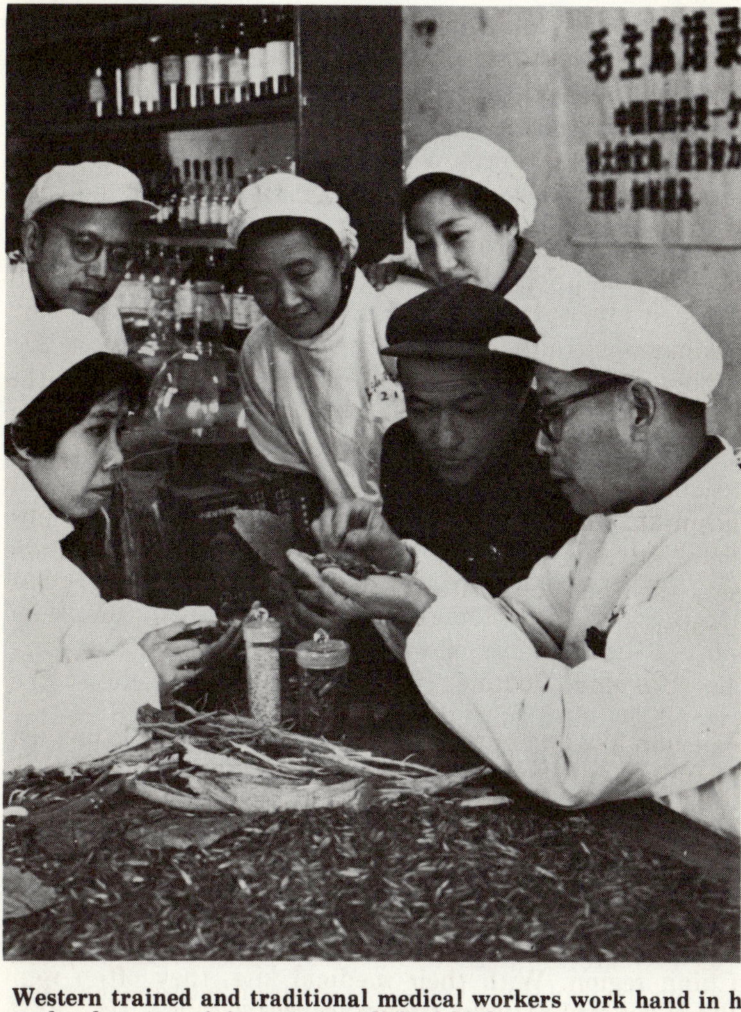

Western trained and traditional medical workers work hand in hand with each other, examining some medicinal herb.

5. Production of Herbal Drugs

As a result of active scientific research on recipes and prescriptions of medicinal herbs, production of drugs from medicinal herbs and from both herbal and Western medicine has gone up rapidly. Many places have tapped the rich resources of inexpensive traditional crude drugs and made various kinds of medicines. On the other hand, there has been a great increase in the output of medicinal herbs and crude drugs, which is made successful by the transplanting and discovering of medicinal herbs. In the catalogue of "Chinese Herbal Drugs," June, 1971, compiled by Chinese Drugs Wholesaler in Hong Kong, several hundred items were listed, together with their ingredients and uses.

6. Miraculous Results

The following table gives some examples resulting from the combined medicine.

7. Serving the People

The special feature of this new system is to serve the people. The patient will not suspect the doctor of being after his money or of using him as a guinea pig. This new voluntary system of medicine, runs on the principle of mutual aid. Commune members pay a small fee every year. This plus funds from the commune make the cooperative medical fund. Treatment requires only a tiny registration fee and medicines are free. The doctor can be honest with the patient, and not perform needless operations, or prescribe unnecessary drugs, or make useless tests. The required treatment, be it traditional or Western, will be done without hesitation and according to the patient.

It is regrettable that the great majority of Western doctors have placed themselves in position that does not

THE "LIMITS" SET BY WESTERN MEDICAL AUTHORITIES	THE ACTUAL PRACTICE OF COMBINED MEDICINE
Limbs completely severed for six hours can be reattached, but may not be functional.	Limbs completely severed for 24 hours are successfully rejoined, and with normal function.
Burns over more than 80% of the body are fatal.	A female worker with over 98% of her body burned was saved. Then her skin was grafted with a new skin.
A heart which has stopped beating for six minutes cannot be revived.	A soldier whose heart "stopped beating" for three hours and twenty-three minutes was saved after an electric shock. And after nine days of continuous medical treatment, he was restored to health.
The after-effects of polio are incurable.	New acupuncture makes people who have been paralyzed for years, stand up and walk again.
Deafness and mutism are incurable.	New acupuncture enables cures for deafness and mutism.
Anesthesia is by conventional method.	New acupuncture enables anesthesia for surgical operations.
Western drugs often fail to stop the continual heavy sweat of a patient recovering from pneumonia.	One dose of an herb drink stops the sweat on the same day.
Pneumonia developing from measles is a dangerous complication. Western medicine alone proved ineffective.	The Chinese traditional treatment is to prescribe medicine that induces full eruption of rash to "bring out the poison." This has proved to reduce complications.
Western fracture treatment gives careful attention to accurate reduction.	The new method adopts accurate reduction and the patient is given both herb medicine and Western drugs. Poultices made from herbs are applied over the fracture. More than 1,800 fracture patients under this treatment recovered in one-third less time than those treated by only Western or traditional method.

recognize traditional Chinese medicine, whereas in China there is no reluctance to adopt the new instruments and techniques of the Western medicine and combine both in patient care.

"This is the hour," said President Nixon, offering his toast at the Welcome Banquet in China. "This is the day for our two peoples to rise to the heights of greatness which can build a new and better world." It is indeed the right time to undertake the project. The day will be coming when we may have one medicine, embodying the best of both cultures.

Chapter 2

Acupuncture Therapy

Acupuncture Therapy

The Western world knew little of traditional Chinese medicine until the 17th century, when Louis the 14th sent to Peking a scientific mission of missionaries to China. These Jesuits who studied the institutions of Chinese civilization and medicine returned to Europe and reported their discoveries. It was they who first coined the word "acupuncture" that comes from two Latin words "acus" and "punctura". Acus means needle; punctura means pricking. It describes this ancient Chinese method of healing. In the Chinese sense, it embodies two treatments: needling and moxibustion. They can be applied together or separately.

2.1 ORIGIN OF ACUPUNCTURE

The origin of acupuncture is shrouded in antiquity. According to tradition, some 5000 years ago, the Chinese noticed that pain could be relieved when they rubbed stones against their bodies. It was also discovered that some soldiers, wounded by arrows, recovered from long suffered illness. This collection of ideas led to the principle that needles inserted into various points of the body, when manipulated, could benefit many diseases. This can be said to be the beginning of acupuncture. The earliest record of an effective cure of a typical case by acupuncture is found in one of the historical records written about 2000 years ago. The book recorded how Pien Chuch (407 B.C - 310 B.C.) the first acupuncture doctor cured a seriously ill prince.

The first text on acupuncture is "The Yellow Emperor's Classic on Internal Medicine" which is dated at about 250

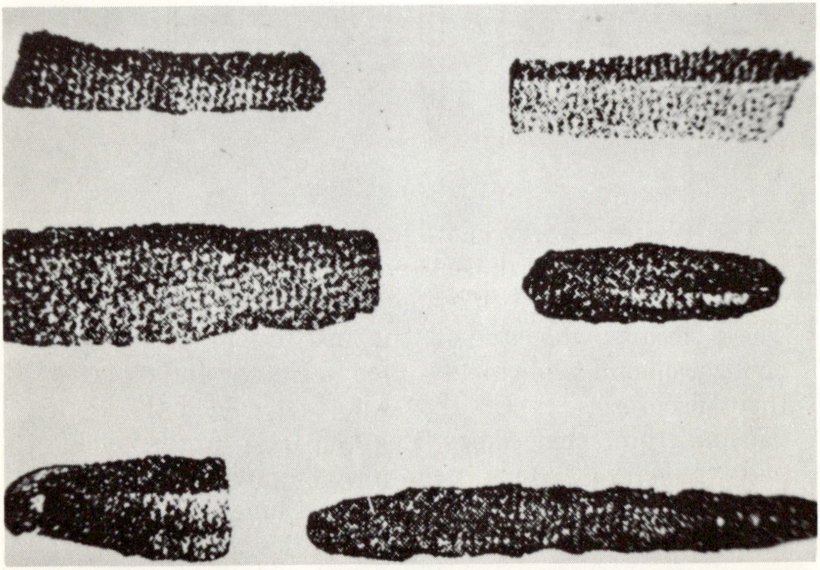

Sharp stones were used as healing instruments in Shang Dynasty (1783-1122 B.C.)— the beginning of acupuncture. *(History of Chinese Medical Science, C. Y. Chen, Chinese Medical Institute, Hong Kong.)*

B.C. It is not only the first medical book in Chinese, but also the oldest medical publication in the world. The entire text is presented in the form of a dialogue between the Yellow Emperor and his ministers. The book is composed of two sections: Su Wan and Ling Shu. Described in the second section is the meridian system, the 132 acupuncture points, different kinds of needles and treatments of diseases. This provides the mystical rationale for the procedure known as acupuncture as practiced in traditional Chinese medicine today.

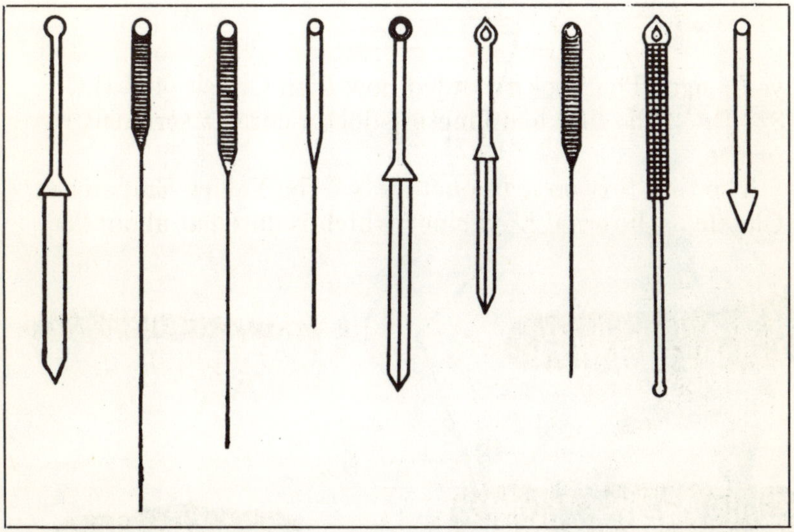

Nine kinds of acupuncture needles were mentioned in "The Yellow Emperor's Classic on Internal Medicine."

In the Sung Dynasty (960 - 1279), acupuncture was fairly popular, Two bronze figures and illustrated documents were made for the sake of acupuncture practice and teaching. The interiors of the bronze statues were filled with models of organs and viscera, while the surfaces were covered with yellow wax and water. Only when inserting the needles into the correct acupuncture point would water gush out.

足少陰腎經之圖

凡二十七穴
左右共五十四穴

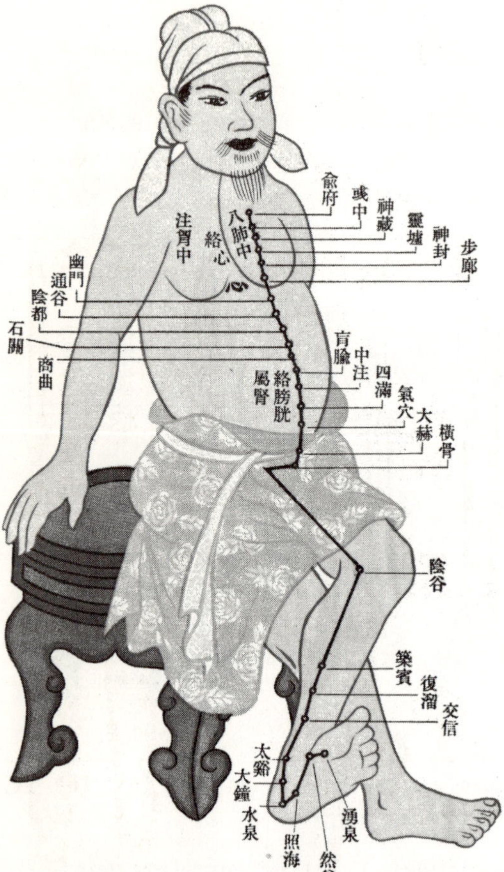

圖五十九——仿明版古圖(五)

Kidneys meridian as shown in ancient medical treatise.

In the past decade there have been many innovations in acupuncture, beginning with the cure of the deaf and mute, the later use of electro-acupuncture, and now more recently the use of acupuncture anesthesia for surgical operations.

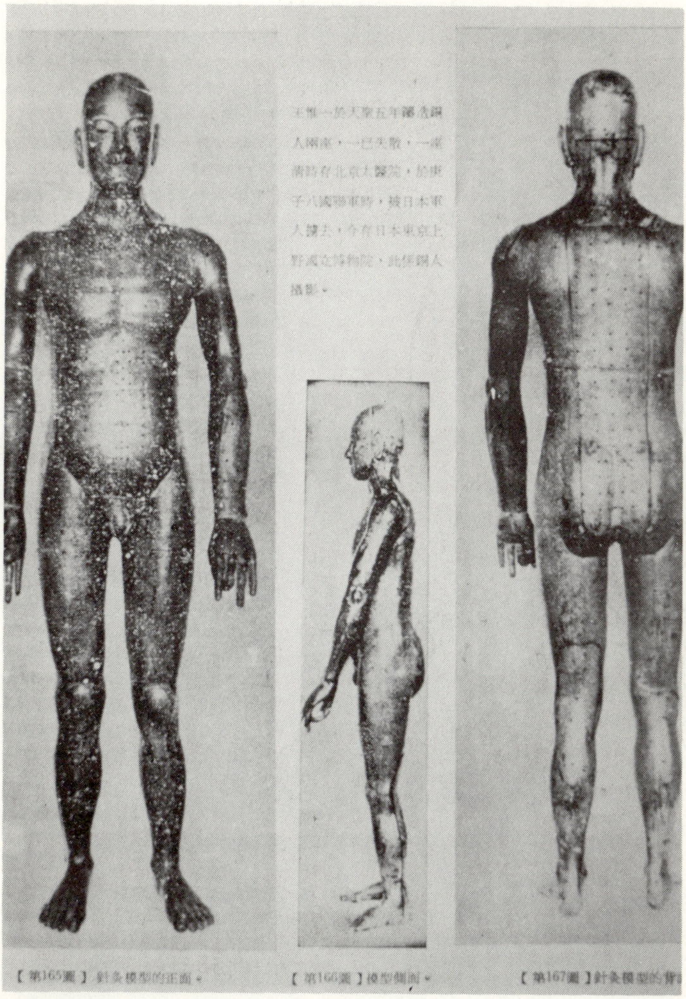

Different views of the first bronze figure—cast in 1026 A.D. *(History of Chinese Medical Science, C. Y. Chen, Chinese Medical Institute, Hong Kong.)*

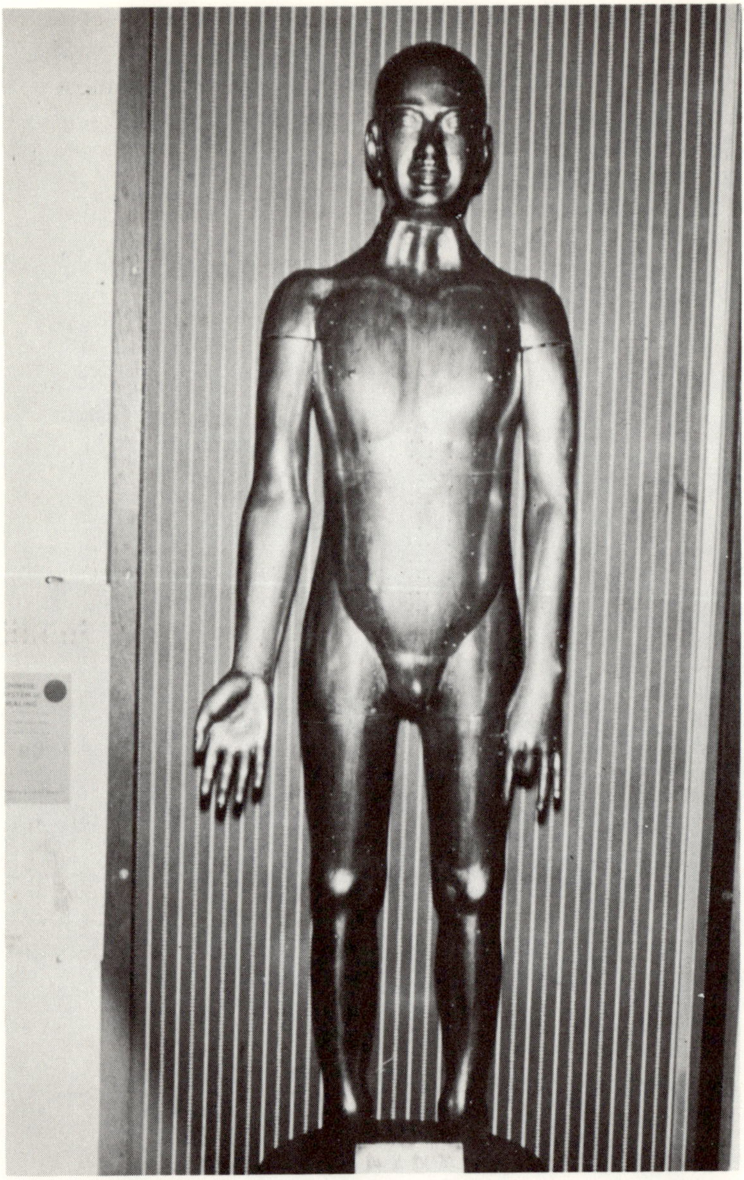

Later model of the bronze figure.

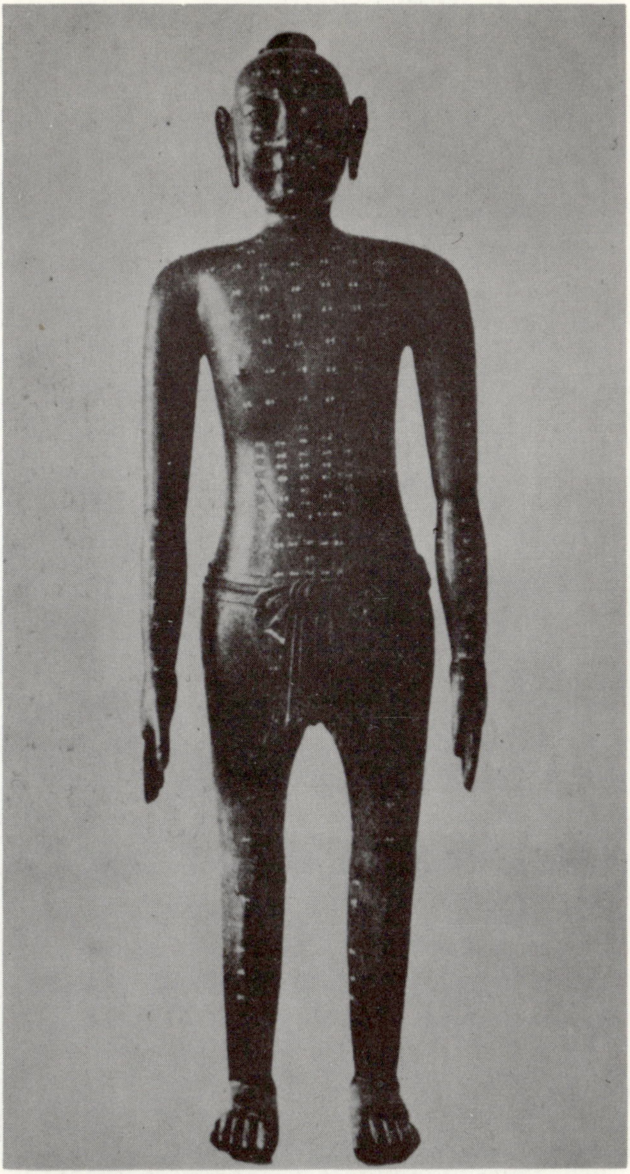

Later model of the bronze figure.

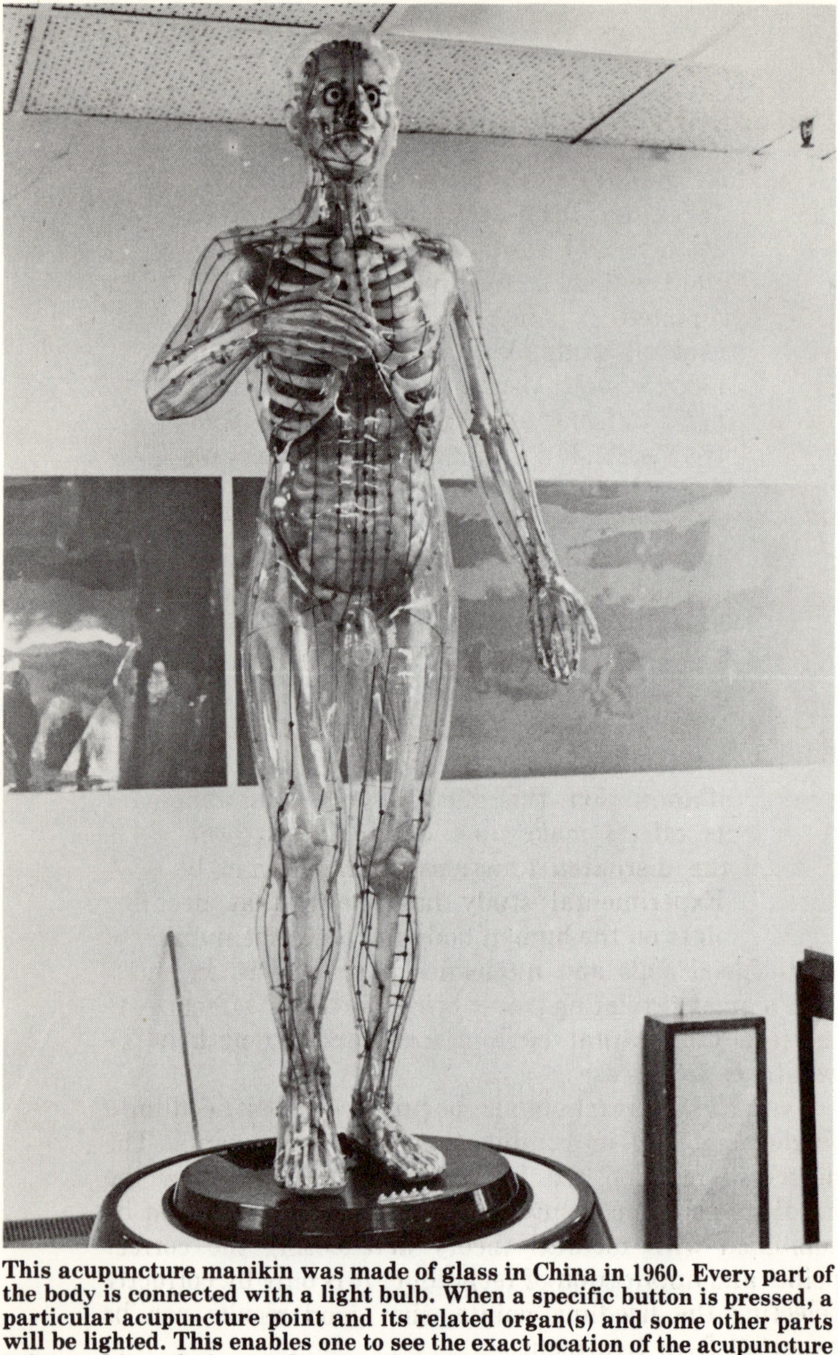

This acupuncture manikin was made of glass in China in 1960. Every part of the body is connected with a light bulb. When a specific button is pressed, a particular acupuncture point and its related organ(s) and some other parts will be lighted. This enables one to see the exact location of the acupuncture point and its relation to the rest of the body.

2.2 NEEDLING

The first needles were made of stone, then it was changed to animal bone and horn, bamboo, iron, gold, silver, steel and now stainless steel. Needles are to be inserted into the body at specific points. These points are called acupuncture points, which are usually located between skeletal joints. Very rarely do they fall on the bones or blood vessels. Usually, a skillful practitioner can use his fingers to feel the exact position of the point when inserting the needle. It does not cause any pain or bleeding.

The needles themselves do not cure, but it is the effect which they produce on the body that is important. The effects of the needling are excitation, inhibition, and induction, which can accordingly affect heart beat, blood count, blood flow, hormone secretion, etc. Excitation means moderate stimulation being applied to activate the function of specific organs, while inhibition seeks to sedate those overly active nerves or glands. If a needle is at a point away from the affected area to induce removal of congestion or inflammation, this effect is called induction. All these three effects make up the regulation power which restores the disrupted functions of the human body to normal. Experimental study has shown that needling certain points on the human body increases the number of white blood cells and intensifies phagocytosis. In short, such a great regulating power brings forth two effects — to increase the natural healing force and strengthen the resistance to diseases.

Two different reactions can be produced when needling a single point and its combination with other points. The degree of reaction can be varied according to how the needle is being manipulated. Clinical experience must be combined with medical theory in choosing the correct points and application of technique. It is only by correctly selecting the needling points, that good results can be expected from treatment.

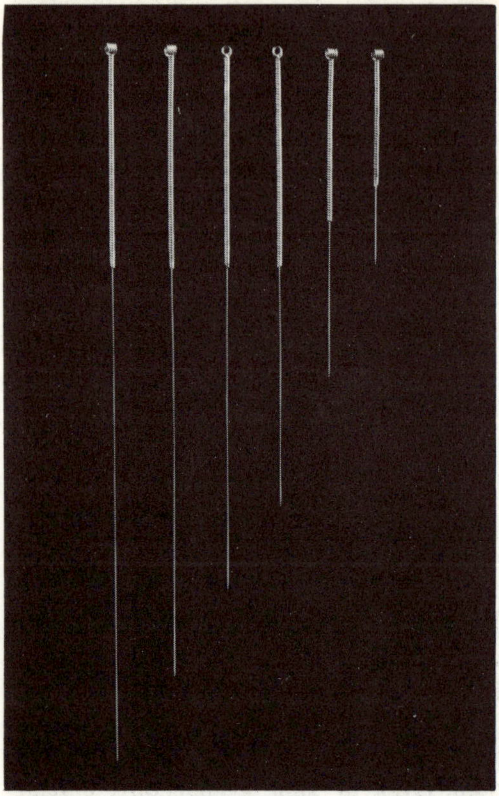

Different lengths of slim acupuncture needles.

The needle is inserted with a quick jab against a stretched or depressed skin surface. The needles that are used for insertion are very fine being of 26 to 32 gauge stainless steel so that they cause the patient little if any pain and very rarely any bleeding.

The needle depth varies from one-half inch to three inches in the body and extremity with the exception of the head where the needles can be inserted less than one-half inch because of the skeletal formation. In the application of needling to the meridians of the body, specific attention must be given to the correct needling points and the position of the instrument as well as great care, avoiding

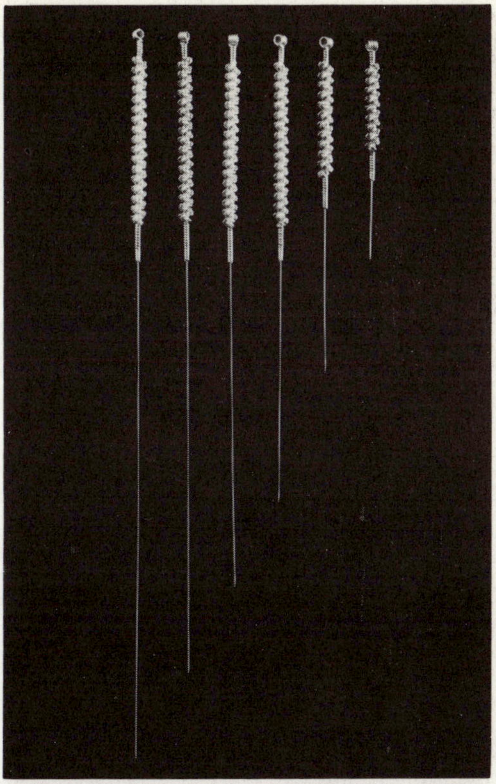

Two types of slim acupuncture needles. Usually from ½" to 3".

the forbidden points in each meridian that are not to be used for either acupuncture and/or moxibustion.

There are nine types of needles mentioned in the ancient Chinese medical treatise, but today, some of them are no longer in use. One will find the following types of needles are those needles commonly used:

1)Slim needles,

This type is the one most commonly used. The shaft usually ranges from one to three inches in length. The hub of the needle which is prepared for manipulation can be varied according to the practitioner's need.

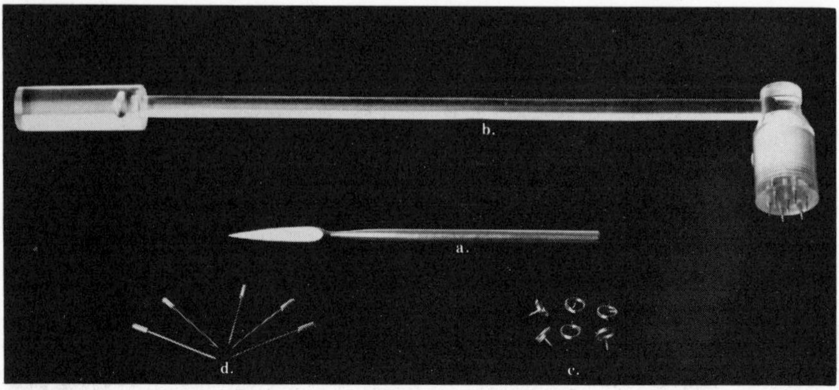

Other acupuncture needles: a) prismatic needle; b) 7-star needle; c) press needle and d) inner dermal needle.

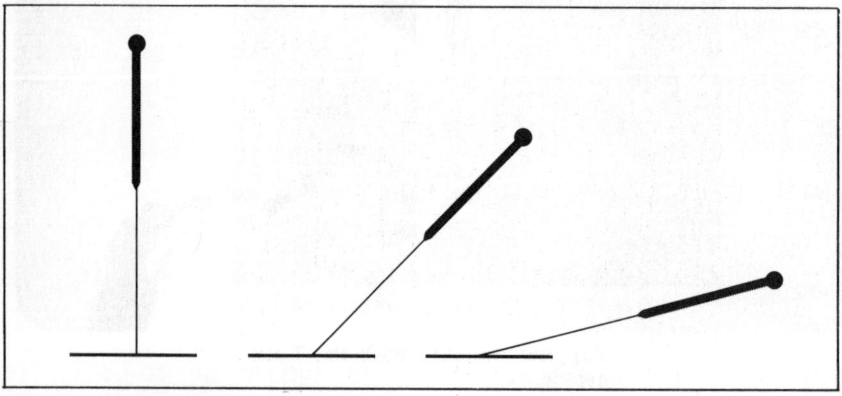

There are 3 ways of inserting the needle: perpendicular to the skin surface, or at an angle of about 45 degrees, or along the skin surface.

2) Prismatic needles,

They are about two and a half inch long with a sharp head; they are good for acute diseases and minor bleeding. Because of its relative large diameter, the insertion should not be more than one-tenth of an inch.

3) 7-star needles,

These are seven or five needles put together and used for hammering over the skin surface. They are especially good for skin diseases and children.

4) Inner dermal needles,

They are rather delicate and good for applying to acupuncture points of the head or ear.

5) Press needles,

They are designed for staying in the skin, usually for one or two days; they are good for chronic disorders of internal organs.

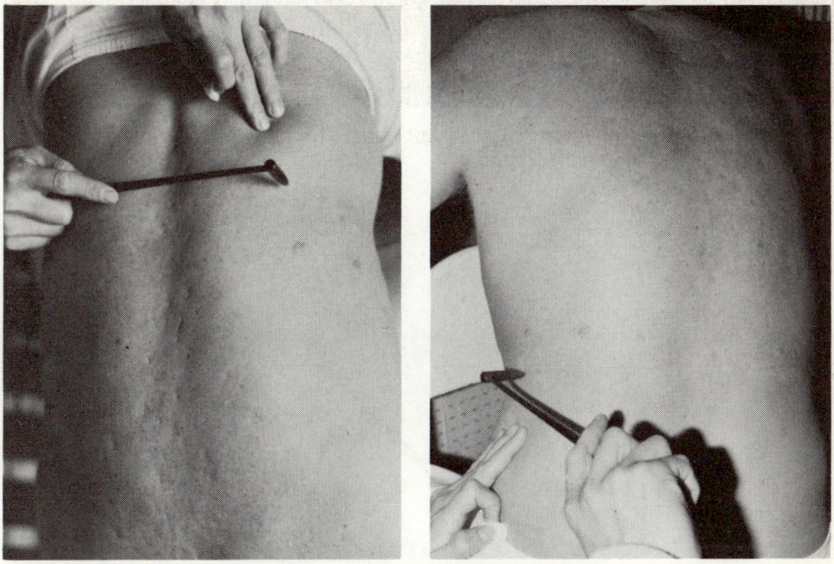

Tapping the skin with the 7-star needle.

2.3 MOXIBUSTION

The buring of moxa, a medicinal herb on or near the skin constitutes another part of acupuncture called "moxibustion". This may be done by applying a small cone of moxa, with or without a slice of ginger, over the acupuncture point. The cone is then ignited and burned down to the skin until a small blister arises. Because of the risk of burnt scars, the moxa may be rolled into a cigar-like shape, ignited and moved around the needles. The distance between the glowing end of the moxa cigar and the skin

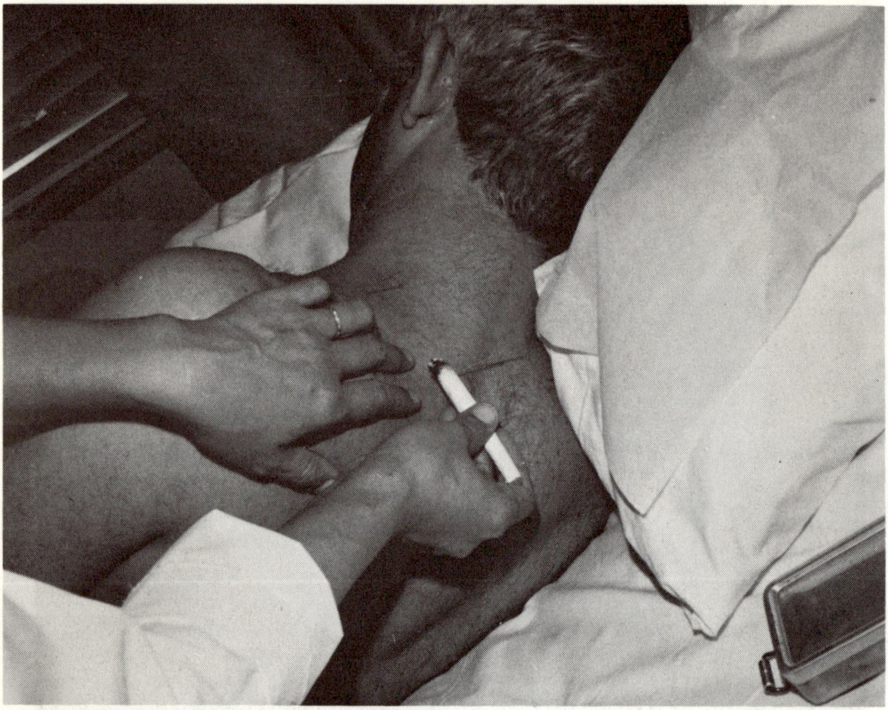

Acupuncture: needling and moxibustion.

surface should be such that the patient can only feel a comfortable warmth. Traditionally, certain sites are prohibited for moxibustion. The effects of moxibustion are to stimulate body functions, such as dilation of blood vessels, stimulation of blood circulation, and acceleration of metabolism. Moxibustion is excellent for certain symptoms such as asthma, anemia, etc. There are several kinds of moxa, but the wooly substance of the Chinese dry wormwood leaves is usually used because of its softness, pleasant smell and gentle heat.

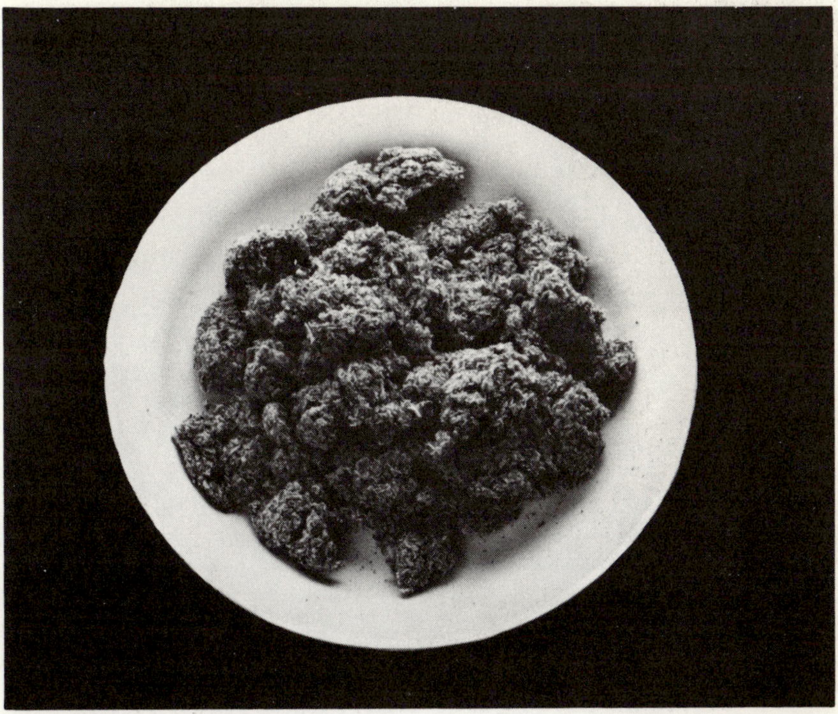

Moxa-dry wormwood leaves.

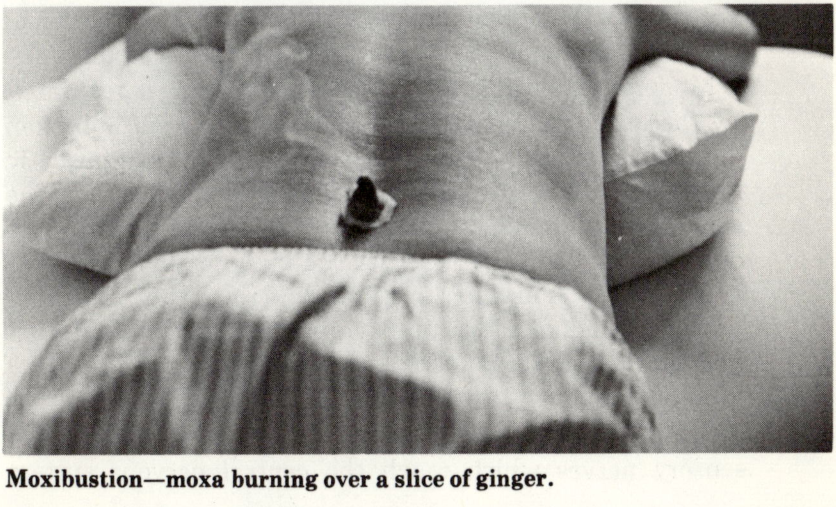

Moxibustion—moxa burning over a slice of ginger.

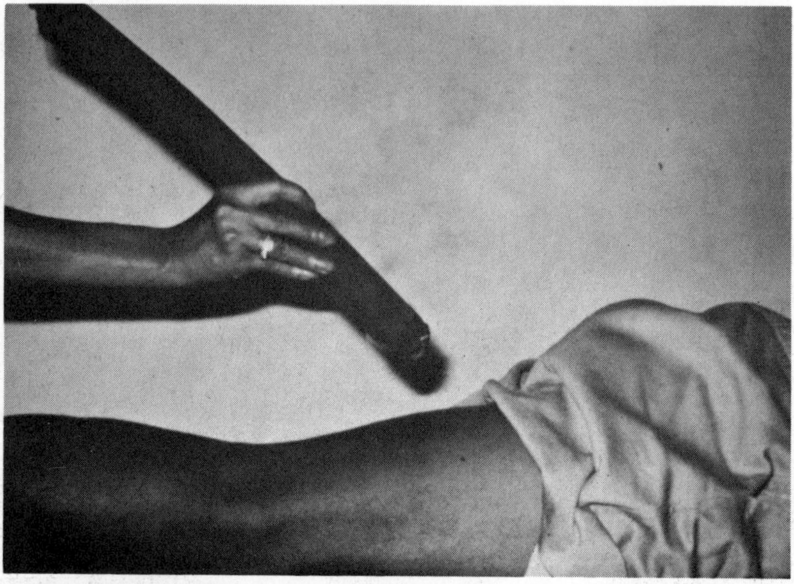

Moxibustion—with a big moxa roll.

2.4 THE TWO DIFFERENT VIEWS OF ACUPUNCTURE—NERVES vs MERIDIANS

The relative specifics of points reflect the fact that there are certain special connections between different parts of the body. But how are these connections affected?

Modern physiology postulates that the body is regulated by the autonomic nervous system. This system is broken down into two separate categories. The para-sympathetic nervous system and the sympathetic nervous system. The general application of these two separate systems are opposing and in general affect the body in that the para-sympathetic nervous system controls the digestive processes and balances the sympathetic nerve excitation and the sympathetic nervous system prepares the body for "fight or flight".

Stimuli may arise from the periphery by collection from sensory nerves which reach the central nervous system

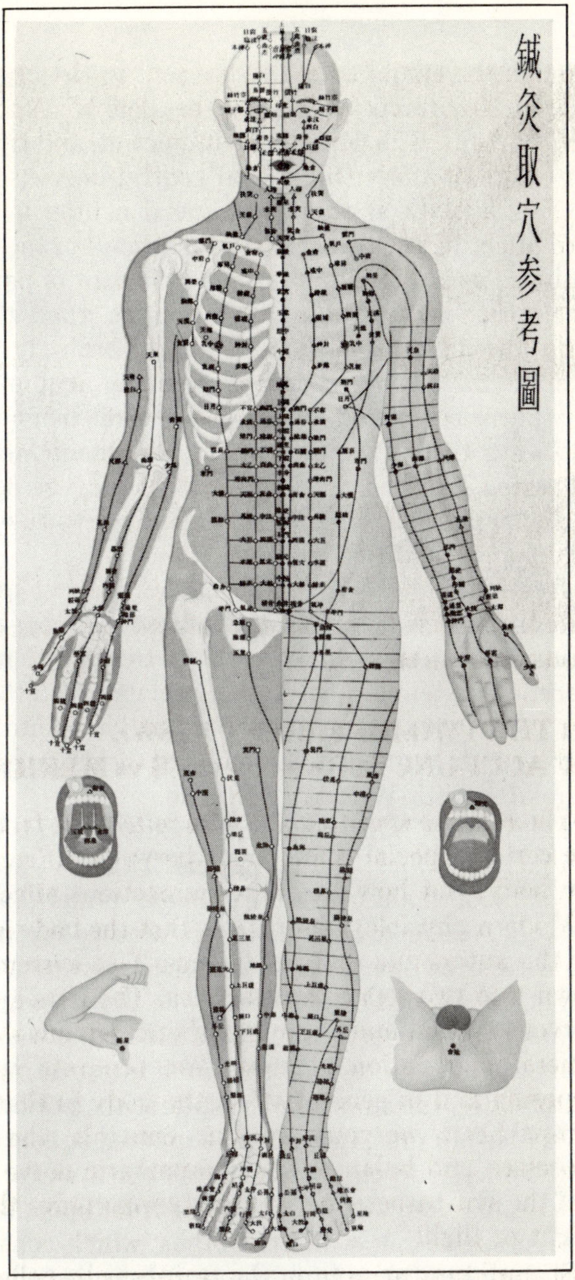

Modern chart showing courses of meridians and acupuncture points.

through the spinal cord and are sent to the brain through appropriate tracts to adjust the body's response to its environment. The points of acupuncture and the meridian system may affect the known central nervous system by causing a block at the intranuncial neuron in the spinal cord affecting the transmission of stimuli to the brain. The pathway would eliminate the recruitment of pain fibers or block the peripheral stimulation so that the painful stimulus cannot be appreciated in the brain. It can be seen that the meridian system and points of acupuncture have not been correlated with the central nervous system pathways that are known in Western medicine. It can be suggested that the meridian system may be a correlated and effective part of the autonomic nervous system that may supply additional information.

There cannot be a simple explanation of exactly how acupuncture may affect the central nervous system in terms of Western medicine because the traditional Chinese meridian system has not been correlated with the accepted central nervous system distribution. The meridian system and acupuncture points have not been investigated or correlated with Western medicine.

Traditional Chinese medicine holds that this connection is affected by means of meridians. This system consists of 12 pairs of main meridians, 2 extra meridians, and a network similar to the human circulatory system. Each of the 12 paired meridians is associated with a particular physiological unit of the body. The units are the 12 basic organs distinguished in Chinese medicine: the lungs, the heart, the large intestine, the small intestine, the kidneys, the bladder, the stomach, the spleen, the pericardium, the tri-heater (an imaginary organ supposed to control Qi), the gallbladder, and the liver. One of the 2 extra meridians, which runs along the middle of the front body, is called the conception vessel; while the other, which runs along the spinal cord to the front of the head is called the governing vessel. The meridian system is to link up all the internal organs and different parts of the body surface, thus making the human body an integrated whole.

2.5 THE ACUPUNCTURE POINTS AND MERIDIANS

According to tradition, there are 365 known vital points, but today some have said there are over a thousand acupuncture points, with about one hundred in common use. Some of them fall in the courses of meridians, while others do not. Some British and French acupuncturists believe that the courses of meridians correspond to the lines of embryological development.

In 1962, Dr. Bongham Kim of North Korea claimed to have identified the anatomical configuration of an acupuncture point and its meridian, called Bongham Corpuscle and Bongham duct as in honor of its discoverer. The Bongham corpuscle consists of groups of small oval cells, surrounded by capillaries, located in the skin, close to the internal organs, blood vessels and lymphatic vessels.

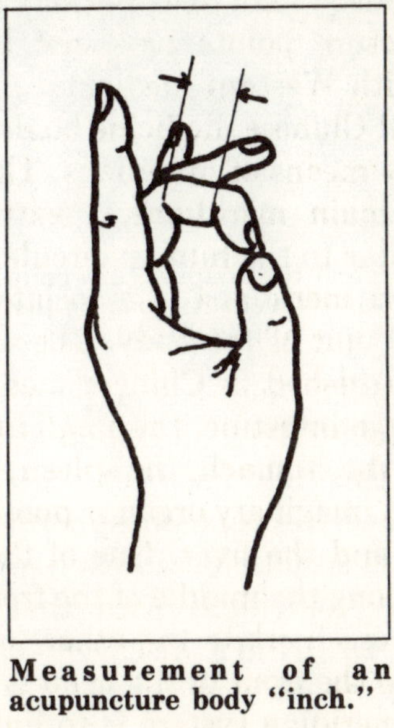

Measurement of an acupuncture body "inch."

These oval cells are different in structure from those of a lymph nodule or blood vessel or nerve fiber. The links between the Bongham corpuscles are named Bongham ducts. They are also different from any other known ducts or tubes such as capillaries, lymphatic glands, etc. Dr. Kim's experiments (used microtomy and staining) to show that these ducts contain a free (uni-directional) flow of some fluid, actuated by the heart. The fluid is pale,

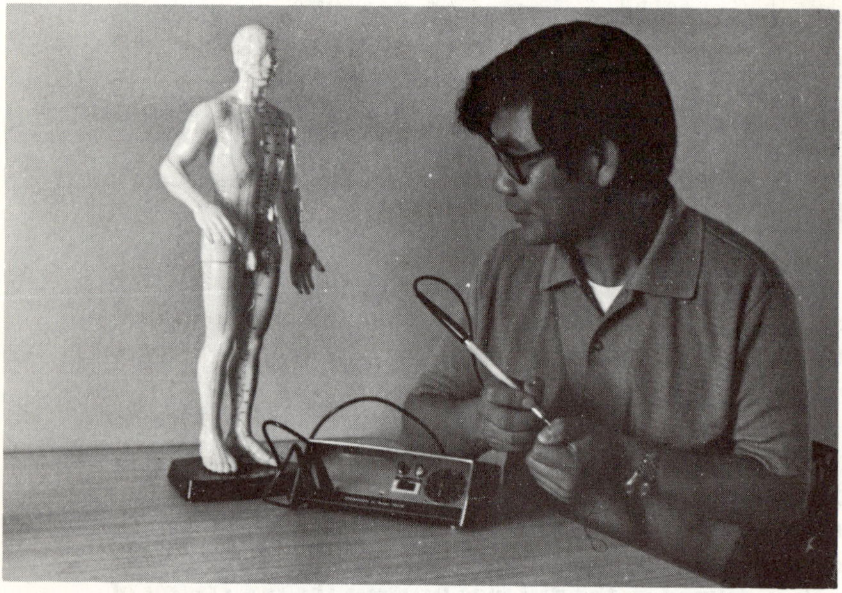

An electronic device to detect the acupuncture point. There are two control lights; one red and the other green. As soon as the needle electrode makes contact with a point, the green light illuminates.

colorless, acellular and has a large quantity of desoxyribonucleic acid (DNA) and ribonucleic acid (RNA). The circulation of this fluid has been ascertained by the aid of radioactive traces (isotope phosphorus 32). When injected into a Bongham corpuscle, radioactive phosphorus traces a path which is coincident with that of the traditional meridians. If Dr. Kim's discovery can be verified, the whole present anatomical knowledge and physiological

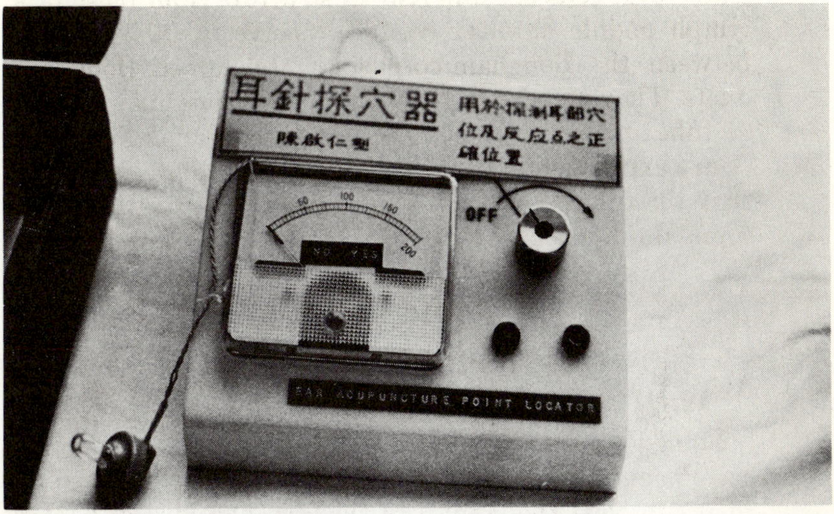

Ear acupuncture point locator.

concepts of Western medicine would undergo a radical change to incorporate another section of the nervous system.

Traditionally, the site of an acupuncture point is measured with reference to the anatomical location. Every part of the human body is divided into units, called acupuncture body "inch". This "inch" is not the same inch as in the English measuring unit. An acupuncture body inch is defined as the distance between the two creases of the phalange, of the bent middle finger. Since we are all of different sizes, the measurement is taken according to the individual.

Acupuncture points have electrical properties. Reduced impedance (resistance and reactance) and higher potential with respects to the adjacent skin surface are found at the acupuncture points. By measuring vicinities of acupuncture points the exact sites can be detected. Such an electronic device is called an acusometer*. The location involves the detection of impedance or potential change between two electrodes on the subject. Usually, the im-

Also known as a stigmascope in France and tobiscope in Russia.

pedance is measured. One electrode, called the indifferent electrode, is grasped by the hand, the other, called the point electrode, is held against the skin surface. The range of impedance encountered in normal surface is from 20,000 ohms to about 200,000 ohms. The electrical impedance and potential at acupuncture points vary, while those of normal skin stays fairly constant.

2.6 DISEASES THAT ARE BEST TREATED BY ACUPUNCTURE

Some Western physicians suggest that acupuncture may be of benefit only in those diseases that are psychosomatic in origin, but the American doctors who visited China, seem convinced that it is impossible to explain acupuncture only in terms of psychosomatics. As a matter of fact, this explanation has been eliminated by Dr. Felix Mann. He has performed acupuncture on patients who have been anesthetized. He found that both the conscious and anesthetized patients have the same satisfactory results. Many people have also advanced terms such as hypnotism, self-suggestion, psychotronics, bioplasics, etc., but none of them gives a satisfactory explanation. The meridian system and acupuncture points can not be easily understood by the Western doctors. But no one can deny that patients are improved or cured of symptoms and an explanation is needed. In some cases, diseases can be effectively treated with acupuncture, where Western medicine is powerless. From an analysis of 213 kinds of diseases suffered by 8,063 patients, it has been shown that the efficacy of acupuncture therapy is as high as 92.5%*.

**The efficacy of acupuncture and Moxibustion", Research Institute of Acupuncture and Moxibustion, Academy of traditional Chinese Medicine, Peking.*

The following list is merely a number of some common examples.

DISEASES	REMARKS
1) Arthritis (all forms) — inflammation of joints. e.g. neuralgia tennis elbow rheumatoid arthritis	It is always related to acupuncture because it is always the only best curative means.
2) Rheumatism — an overall term to cover diseases of muscles, tendon, joint, bones or nerve. e.g. degenerated joint diseases bursitis lumbago myositis	same as arthritis.
3) Gynaecology — female problems. e.g. irregular menstruation scanty menstruation painful menstruation	Excellent. In China, acupuncture is also used for birth control, abortion as well as sterility.
4) Neurology — disorder of the nervous system. e.g. epilepsy hysteria nervousness Sciatica neuralgias paralysis polio	Can be greatly improved. Most of the patients begin to feel an alleviation of pain after three, four, or five treatments.

DISEASES	REMARKS
5) Stomach and intestines troubles. e.g. excessive acidity gastralgia gastritis loss of appetite non-digestion ulcer vomiting	Excellent.
6) Pains of all kinds. e.g. colic headache migraine toothache	Acupuncture is excellent in killing the pain.
7) Infectious diseases e.g. malaria diarrhea dysentery influenza	Good.
8) Deafness and mutism	New acupuncture technique has enabled the deaf to hear and the mute to speak. (please see 2.7 for detail)
9) Others e.g. asthma angina bronchitis high blood pressure insomnia skin diseases	Good.

2.7 TREATING THE DEAF AND MUTE

The following is an account of curing deafness and mutism in an article by Audrey Topping in Vogue, January, 1972. (Reprinted by permission of the Conde Nast Publications, Inc.)

> I visited Number Three School for Deaf-Mutes in Peking and Wang Chen-ying, a member of the school's propaganda team, explained the process of thinking that led to the discovery:

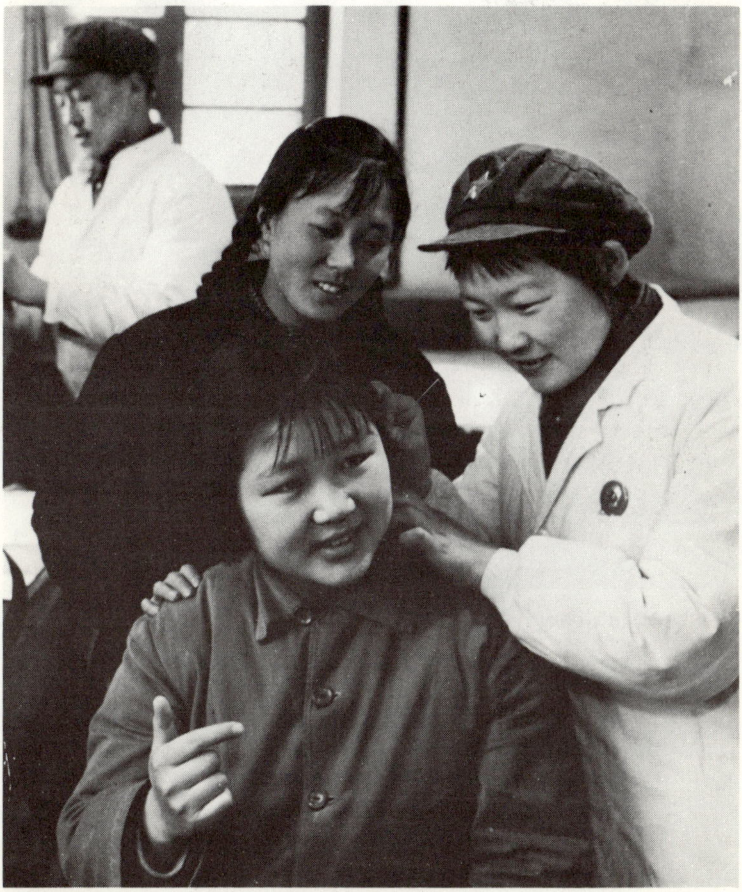

Treating a deaf-mute pupil in Peking, China.

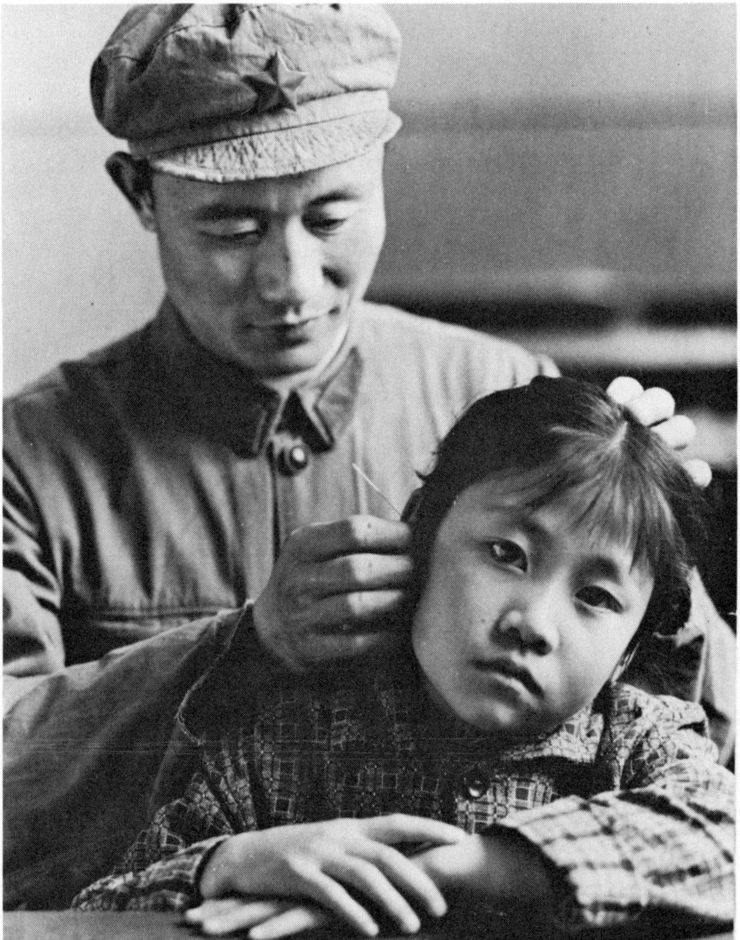

Treating a student in a deaf-mute clinic. *(New China News)*

"Previously doctors said that deafness and dumbness were incurable, but the Red Army medical team has the view that nothing is incurable. We studies Mao's writing on contradictions. He says that in studying any process, if it has more than two contradictions, first find the main one; then proceed. Which is the main contradiction here? In analyses we learned that language is first received through the ears. In case histories we found that most deafness was caused in one- to three-year-olds as a result of a high fever, brain inflammation, or other diseases. This caused deafness and the vocal organs, although they were actually in good condition, degenerated from lack of use into a diseased state. Dumbness was often caused by deafness so this was the first contradiction. To solve this we must cure deafness. Chairman Mao says, "If you want to know the taste of a pear you must eat it." We tried needles on our own bodies to find the proper acupuncture points. We were healthy men and sometimes feared we would injure ourselves, but with Mao's thought, "Everything for the people," in mind we continued the experiments. After repeated trials, we discovered the acupuncture points that cured deafness. Now, after a year's treatment, 90 percent of the afflicted students have a certain capacity for hearing.

"The next contradiction," he went on, "is dumbness. After hearing is recovered, we teach speech. In little more than a year, of our 238 students, eleven have been completely cured and have gone into regular schools."

Miss Yeh Nu-hsu, a bright-eyed sixteen-year-old with long braids, was among the students. My husband and I spoke to her and she said in halting, but clear Chinese, "Until one year and a half ago, I was deaf and mute. Now I can talk and even sing." She was obviously overjoyed by her newly found senses and was one of the better students.

Dr. Fang Chou-suan, an army doctor, took us on a tour of the school where the teachers spoke warmly of the importance of encouraging each child individually.

The classes divide into four main categories. First, classes for new students where finger language is used and charts explain the treatment in store for the children. The second category includes acupuncture treatments and tests hearing nerves for response. Third, students are taught the basic sounds; and, fourth, they are taught to speak in special language classes with mathematics, science and history added in the latter two categories — students being encouraged to reply orally.

In the acupuncture room the teacher and an army medical aide insert long needles near the ears and into the arms of the children in what appears to be a painless procedure. The needle is twisted by hand until the nerve is stimulated and the child utters a small cry.

The students first undergo a ten-day course of treatment and then rest for seven days. For the first course there is a special set of points. Then a check of the progress report, and another set, depending on the results, is plotted for the second course.

"Acupuncture spurs the nerve system and adjusts the hearing nerve," Dr. Fang said. "We use several points. The acupuncture points near the ears have quick but temporary effects while the points farther away, as in the arms and hands, have a slower but permanent effect." Some students react quickly, show good results in six months, but most cases take about a year. Deafness caused by brain injury or inflammation is more difficult to deal with. The aim is to get the child to hear from a distance of three meters and to carry on until the hearing reaches twenty meters. Then acupuncture is stopped and concentration on teaching speech begins. The younger the student, the more effective the treatment in most cases.

2.8 FRIENDS OF ACUPUNCTURE

The following people are just some of those prominent figures in the world who have been successfully treated by acupuncture.

Prince Bernhard of The Netherlands recovered from pain in his back, left shoulder and arm which dated from a 1937 automobile accident. Being afflicted again, but diagnosed as constipation problem, the patient was treated for another two days. Then he, at the age of 60, proclaimed that he felt ten years younger.

Premier Lon Nol of Cambodia had great improvement on his massive stroke

James Reston, columnist and vice president of New York Times, had acupuncture to relieve the pressure and distension of the stomach after his emergency operation of appendicitis.

The late President John Kennedy of the United States, Sir Winston Churchill, former Prime Minister of England, Aldous Huxley, the famous writer, and former Indonesian President Sukarno, have all been benefited from treatment of acupuncture.

Tung Pi-wu, now Acting Chairman of the People's Republic of China, 1950 once suffered from pain in the bladder, rendering movement painful. This persisted for several years, despite many attempts at healing. Later when he was treated by acupuncture, his bladder recovered. In his preface to an acupuncture book published in 1954, Peking, he said, "Acupuncture therapy has enjoyed a long history in Chinese medicine. It has been recorded in the oldest medical treatises. Throughout all ages, acupuncture has been practiced in both towns and villages. For certain diseases, there are no drugs required and yet they are often cured. Indeed, the efficacy and speed in healing of acupuncture are often astonishing. This is especially so since we only know that it works but not why it works, and also the practitioners often treat the science as a secret. Western doctors on the other hand, often regard acupuncture as unscientific and therefore have not seriously considered the practice of acupuncture. Therefore, although acupuncture is now in common use in China, it is still locked by a veil of mystique. It would be a great boom to medical science if acupuncture could be studied scientifically, in order to understand the principles and to improve and increase its uses. In China, where both drugs and medical workers are lacking, it is especially important to develop and spread the use of acupuncture, a science indigenous to the working people......." Mao Tse-tung, Chairman of Communist Party of the People's Republic of China, has said, "Chinese medicine and pharmacology are a great treasure house and effects should be made to explore them and raise them to a higher level."

2.9 SOME HISTORICAL CASES OF ACUPUNCTURE

The reader may find the following historical cases interesting, yet unbelievable, and thus will inevitably consider them as some kind of myth. But believe it or not, these are the actual cases of acupuncture recorded either in the Chinese historical records or ancient writings. As I mentioned before that the first recorded effective cure was by Pien Chuch during the Warring States period (475 - 221 B.C.). Here is how he was described. Pien Chuch once went to a state called Quick. There, he heard about the abrupt death of a prince. Being suspicious, he immediately rushed to the palace and inquired about the matter. After a careful analysis of all the symptoms and the history of the "dead" prince, he said with confidence that the prince might be saved and he was ready for the cure. He was then led to see the "dead" prince. As Pien Chueh carefully examined the body, he found that the prince still had a very weak breath and also the muscle between the two thighs was not cold at all. Therefore, he pronounced the prince was not dead, but actually in a serious state of coma — loss of consciousness. He then pulled out several needles and inserted them into the prince's head, chest, and limbs. After a while, the prince woke up. Meanwhile, Pien Chuch applied moxibustion around his armpits. A herbal drink was also prepared. The prince gradually got up. After another twenty days, the prince was completely recovered.

2. Empress Chan Sun had conceived a baby (he later became the third emporor (Go Cheung) of Tang dynasty (618 - 907 A.D.) and was ready to deliver. Several days had elapsed, but the baby still stayed in the womb. The emperor (Tai Cheung) was so anxious that he ordered for his own personal physician, Li. After taking the expectant mother's pulse, he concluded that the baby was grasping his mother's heart, so he could not be delivered. The emperor did not know what to do and waited for Li's advice. Li told him that he could either save the baby or the mother. The mother uttered, "Save the baby. Long live the Tang dynasty". Li then used a long needle to pierce through her abdomen, until it reached the baby's hand grasping his mother's heart. Shocked by the pain, the baby promptly released his hand from his mother's heart and was then delivered. The baby was examined and a mark made by the stinging of the needle was found.

3. Once there were a very famous acupuncture doctor — Cheung and his student. One day, the concubine of a duke got an emergency illness. Her husband immediately sent for Cheung, but to find Cheung was out of town. So his student came. After making a diagnosis, the student said the patient was seriously ill, and there was only one acupuncture point that might save her life. He then punctured a needle into the ankle of her foot. Sucked in by the circulation, the needle stayed in the ankle and could not be pulled out. The student was so afraid that he apologized to the duke and said, "I have got the point; but I do not know how to get the needle out. Please send for

my master at once." The duke then sent his servant to get Cheung back. The next day Cheung came. He laughed and said the point was a very good point, but his student had not fully mastered the technique. He then needled a point in the wrist of the patient's hand. As soon as the needle was inserted, the other needle shrouding in the ankle jumped out. The patient then recovered.

4. The following is not related to acupuncture, but the reader may find it worthwhile to note.

There was a rich American merchant by the name of G.M. Gest. He suffered from an eye disease and failed to get a cure, despite all attempts by doctors all over the world. In 1930, he went to Peking, China. There, he was healed by a Chinese herbal drug. Amazed by the wonders of Chinese medicine, he collected 75,000 volumes of Chinese medical books. These books were later donated to Princeton University, where the Gest Oriental Library was formed in 1953 in honor of the donor.

Chapter 3

Electro-acupuncture

Electro-acupuncture

Electro-acupuncture is a new healing science integrating traditional acupuncture with modern technology. Basically, there are two kinds of devices. The first device, dealing with the needling, is called the acupuncture stimulator. It is a device to take over the burden of manual manipulation of the needles. The second one, involving the production of heat, is called the acupuncture heater.

3.1 ACUPUNCTURE STIMULATOR

The stimulator is the principal tool for electro-acupuncture therapy, so a clear understanding of its function is essential to its actual uses. Electro-acupuncture differs from conventional electro-therapy on the ground that they operate on two different principles.

In electro-acupuncture, the needle penetrates into particular human structure and utilizes the electric current as a stimulator, whereas conventional electro-therapy uses surface stimulation or the penetrating heating action of electromagnetic waves.

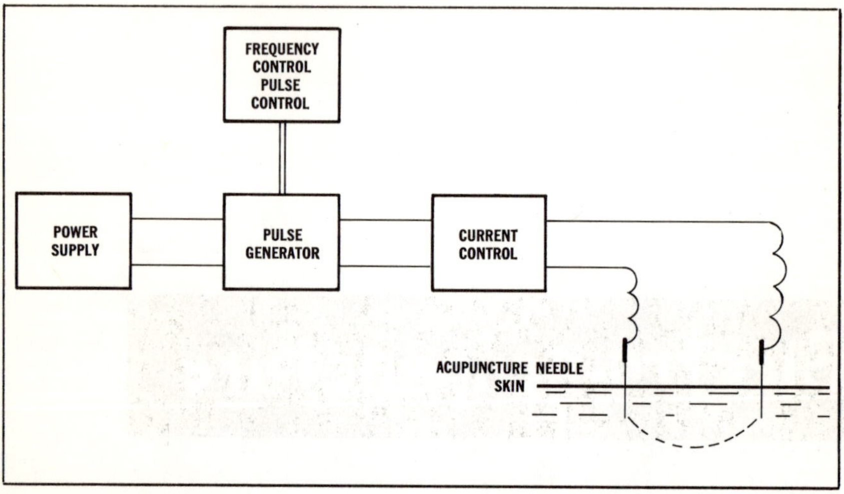

Block diagram showing the design of an acupuncture stimulator.

The most primitive stimulator uses a battery as current source. The needle is inserted into the subject with the positive terminal in contact with the skin and the negative terminal touching the needle for some time.

In recent years, acupuncture stimulators have been greatly improved and, at present, there are many versions of such devices for clinical application. The following types have been used clinically for some time and have been shown to be effective.

1) Battery powered D.C. pulse stimulator.
2) Inductive stimulator.
3) A.C. powered D.C. pulse stimulator.
4) Vacuum-tube oscillator stimulator.
5) Transistorized oscillator stimulator.

All acupuncture stimulators operate on the same principle. First, an electromotive source to drive the machinery — this can be a battery (direct current). Secondly a pulse generator (including frequency and pulse-shaping controls) to vary the nature of the current. There should be a current control to modulate the amplitide of the current.

The stimulator operates in the range of three to twelve volts. In using house current, a transformer is necessary for stepping down the voltage.

The pulse generator causes vibrations in the current of given frequency and shape. The frequency is (?) Hertz (cycles per second) or higher and the pulse shape can be rectangular, sine wave, sawtooth. etc. the last one being the most frequently used. In addition, better devices should have proper pulse durations, usually between 2-6 micro-seconds. Pulse shape is an important determinant of the nature of the stimulator; an inappropriate pulse shape can cause adverse effects.

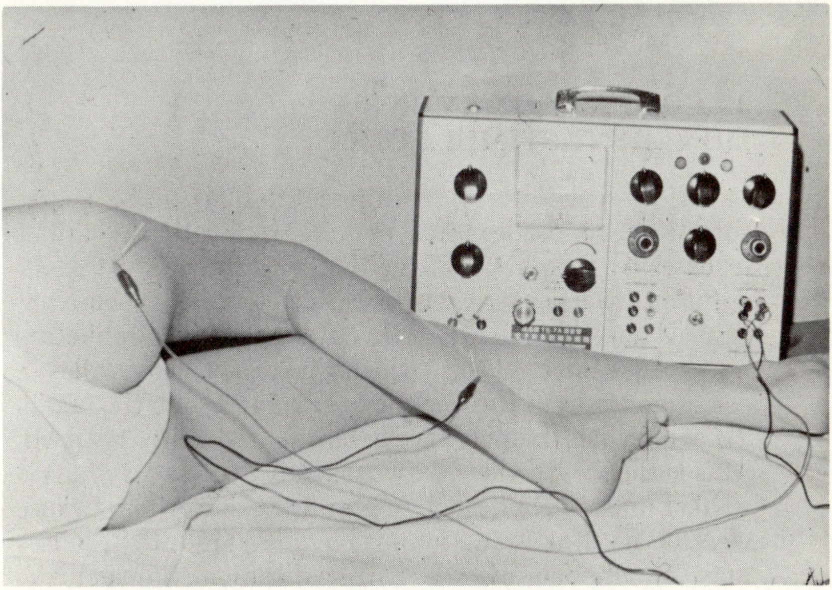

Electro-acupuncture—treating a patient with polio.

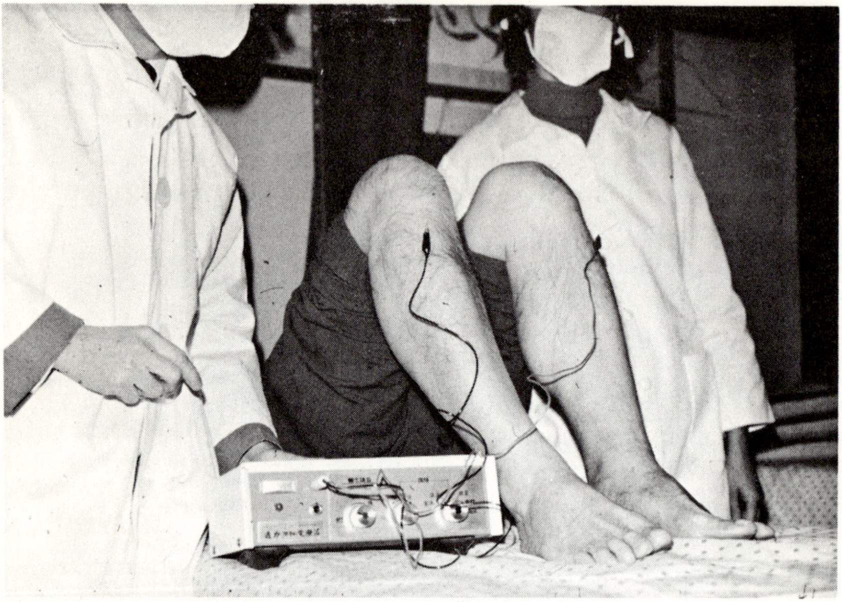

Electro-acupuncture—treating a patient with stomach trouble.

3.2 COMPARISON AMONG DIFFERENT STIMULATORS

Various stimulators have different designs, and of course somewhat properties. For clinical applications, various diseases will require suitable chosen therapy.

Pure D.C. has a strong inhibitive effects and is commonly used for skin diseases. But D.C. electro-acupuncture may cause electrolysis, which in serious cases has a corrosive effect in the body, causing damage to the organ. To avoid this, the polarity should be frequently reversed. This is the most serious drawback. D.C. pulses may have a weaker inhibiting effect than pure D.C., but will not cause electrolysis. If a strong inhibition is required, D.C. pulses may be applied over a longer duration, so that the inhibiting effect accumulates and increases.

The inductive current has a large exciting effect, but its inhibiting effect is inferior to the D.C. pulse. When inductive current is used in electro-acupuncture, strong contractions of the muscle often results, so it has to be applied with the consideration of the state of the disease in mind. The D.C. pulse has a rather smaller exciting effect, but is generally found to be satisfactory.

The vacuum-tube stimulator and the transistor stimulator assemble the D.C. pulse stimulator and have both inhibitive or exciting effects. It is important to get the pulse shape accurate in these machines, for a square wave would be strongly inhibitive.

Clinical experience indicates that most diseases do not require very strong inhibition or excitation and the errors tend more often to be ones of excess. Therefore, the duration, amplitude and the characteristic of the current must be given serious considerations.

As far as mechanical structure is concerned, the pure D.C. case is the simplest. The D.C. pulse stimulator and the inductive stimulator use mechanical vibrations, and often develop complications due to drifts in mechanical characteristics. The vibrating leaf must be of good quality and the contact point should be made of tungsten alloy for durability. The transistor and vacuum tube stimulators have stable oscillations and have a longer life, but the structure is more complicated and a higher cost in construction is to be expected.

For the power source, a battery is certainly simpler, but can not withstand prolonged use. A fairly large battery will last 3-4 hours under continuous use, so in a fixed clinic, house current is more suitable after it is adapted for use.

The D.C. pulse and the inductive stimulators have been clinically tested and used for quite some time and much experience has been gained in their use. The vacuum tube and transistor devices have not been used quite as extensively. However, they apparently have certain characteristics. But medical instruments can not be truly

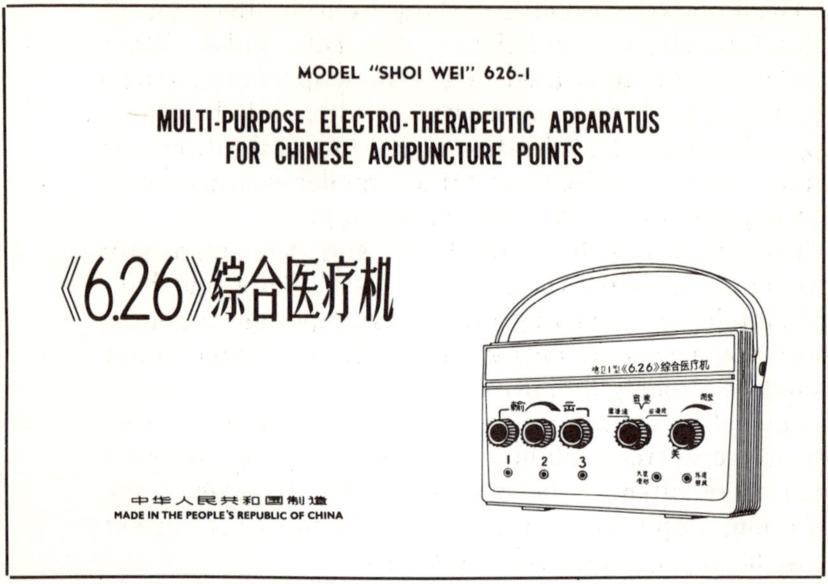

Multi-purpose Electro-therapeutic Apparatus for Chinese Acupuncture Points.

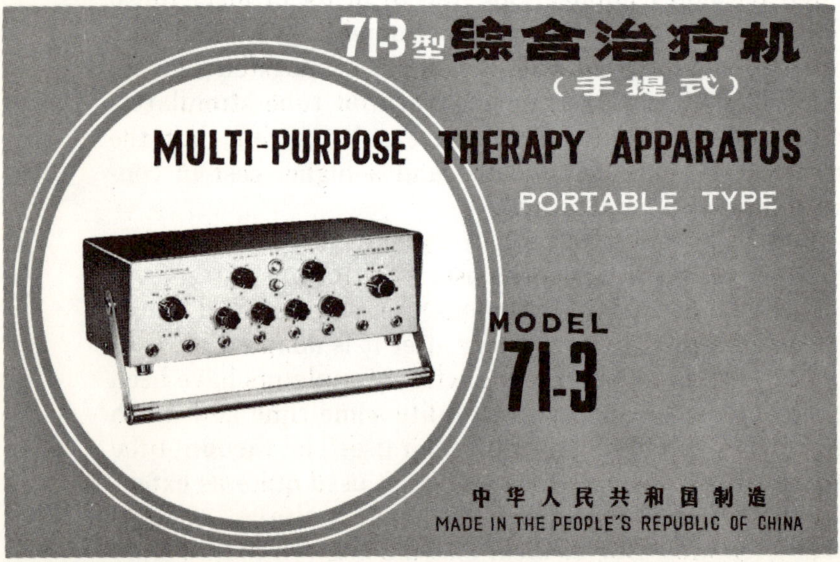

Multi-purpose Therapy apparatus.

evaluated until long-term and wide-range testing and use have verified their capabilities. In any event, the many good features of the vacuum and transistor stimulators will surely increase the healing power of electro-acupuncture. We are now in the age of technology, acupuncture will doubtlessly find a place in the world of electronics.

As of 1972, China has produced 3 types of acupuncture stimulators on the market, namely Model 626-1 Electronic Pulsating Stimulator, Model "Shoi Wei" 626-1 Multi-purpose Electro-therapeutic apparatus for Chinese acupuncture points, and Model 71-3 Multi-purpose Therapy Apparatus. All of them are portable and can apply for treatment as well as anesthesia.

3.3 SOME PRECAUTIONS WHEN USING THE STIMULATOR

To avoid unexpected results from misuse of the stimulator, it is always advisable only for those who are medically qualified workers to perform the treatment on human subjects. But still, there are some steps one must bear in mind before treatment.

1) Check the instrument, see whether it is functioning well. Use a 0-10V voltmeter or a 0-500 micro-amp. ammeter for this purpose. If the indicator of the meter is rising steadily and evenly, it means the stimulator is in good order. If there is no meter at hand, one may test it by putting the 2 electrodes on the tongue. The sensitive feeling of the tongue can tell whether the output of the stimulator is too strong or too weak.

2) When receiving the treatment, the patient should lie on the operating table. The stimulator must be grounded. The operating table must be insulated. This is especially important when using an A.C. current. Thus in case of current leakage, electrical shock hazard can be avoided. Also when operating the stimulator, it is important to start with the weakest current, up to the point the patient feels comfortable, and when cutting off the current, reduce the

current gradually.

3)Always explain to the patient (especially for those who are new to the stimulator) what would happen when treated with the stimulator, such as numbness, soreness, itching, swelling and vibrations. Give the patient a psychological preparation.

4) The patient should be at ease when being treated with the stimulator. Too nervous a patient will cause unexpected or undesirable response.

3.4 ACUPUNCTURE HEATER

As a substitution for the burning of moxa, which provides heat, electric heat is often used. The most common source of heat utilized is infrared rays, which can penetrate deep into the body through the lymphatic system. Effects are similar to, but greater than, the burning of moxa.

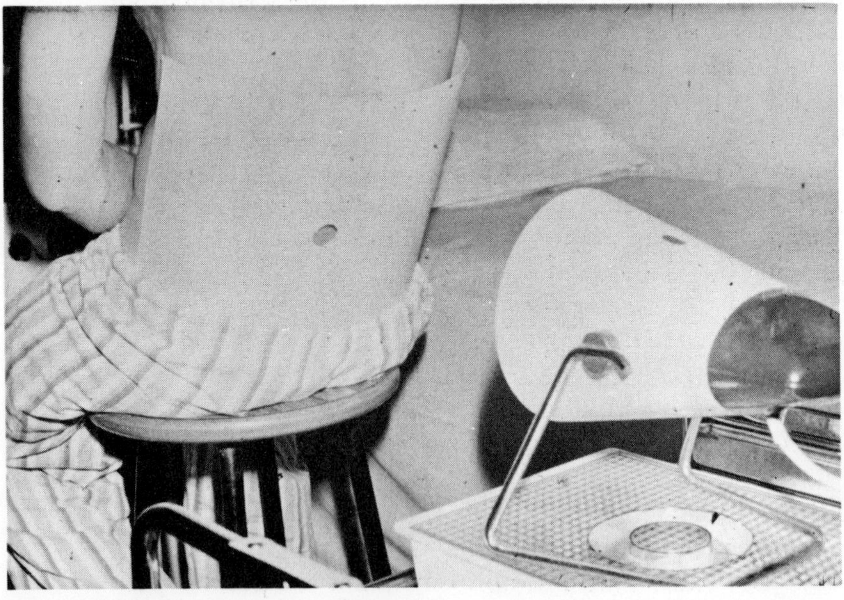

The use of infrared rays for moxibustion.

The distance between the source and skin surface is about 20-40 centimeter. An insulator with a small hole to expose the acupuncture point is used.

Other devices include ultra-violet rays, electric heaters, inspirators, and ultra-sonic waves.

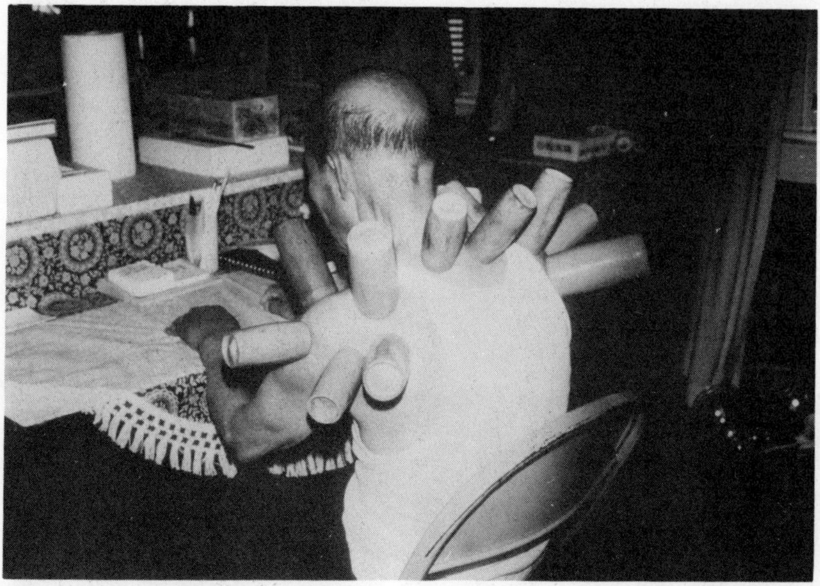

The use of inspirator.

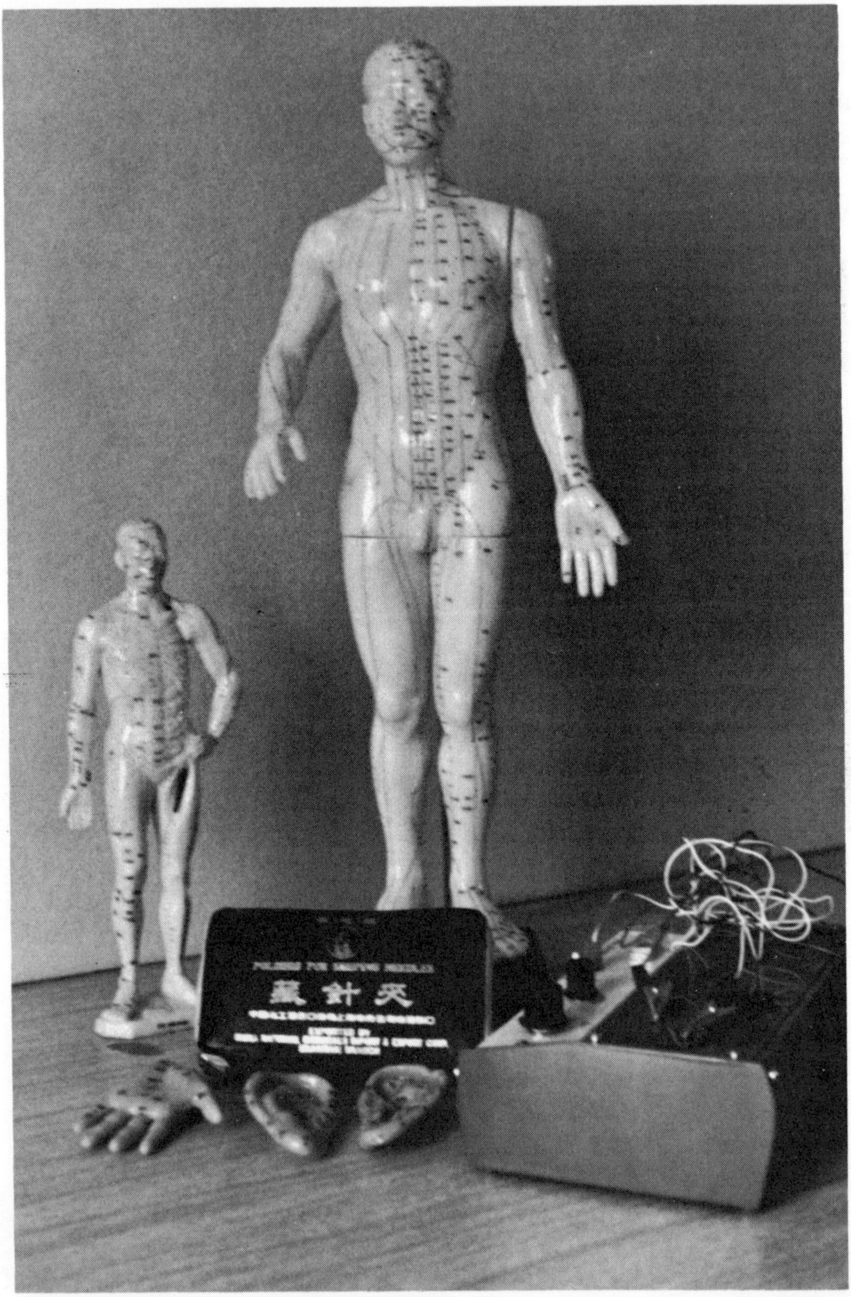

Some acupuncture instruments from China.

Chapter 4

Acupuncture Anesthesia

Acupuncture Anesthesia

During the past few years, the world has heard with astonishment about acupuncture anesthesia. Acupuncture needles are used as the sole anesthetic in surgical operations, while the patients remain awake and pain free. Over half a million operations, including dental, gynecological, gastrectomy, lung, brain, and even brain and open-heart surgeries have been performed. Statistics have shown 75-90% of them successful. The remaining patients required additional anesthetic agents because of a break-through of pain or of insufficient muscle relaxation.

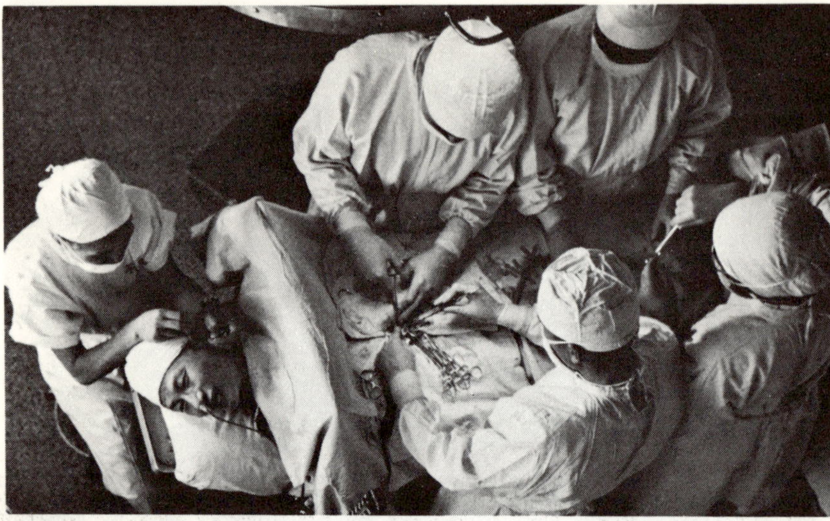

Acupuncture anesthesia is used in the removal of the greater part of a patient's stomach at Peking, China. *(New China News)*

4.1 ORIGIN OF ACUPUNCTURE ANESTHESIA

Since 1958, most of the medical personnel have been trained with Western and traditional Chinese medicines. Acupuncture procedures are being used in all the modern hospitals in China along with Western-style or modern medicines. This is to marshall all medical manpower for two basic missions: to make some sort of care available to the entire population and to drill the people into becoming active participants in public health campaign.

Since pain could be stopped by acupuncture, medical workers at first applied this technique to lessen post-operative pain and achieved satisfactory results. They then thought pain could be prevented if certain acupuncture points were inserted with needles. This gave them the needed inspiration for conducting experiments. From more than 100,000 observations, they found that sensitivity to pain on certain parts of the body was dulled by needling certain distant points. Pain sensation was felt again only after a much stronger stimulus than the original was given.

Acupuncture was found to be effective not only in easing toothache but also in providing anesthesia for tooth extractions. It was then applied to tonsillectomy and other oral-pharyngeal operations. However, it was not widely used until 1966 — an indirect result of the Cultural Revolution in China. Continuous practice in the past few years has helped in perfecting the method of anesthetization by acupuncture. The number of needles have been reduced from 40 to two or three. Manual manipulation of the needles has been replaced by an acupuncture stimulator.

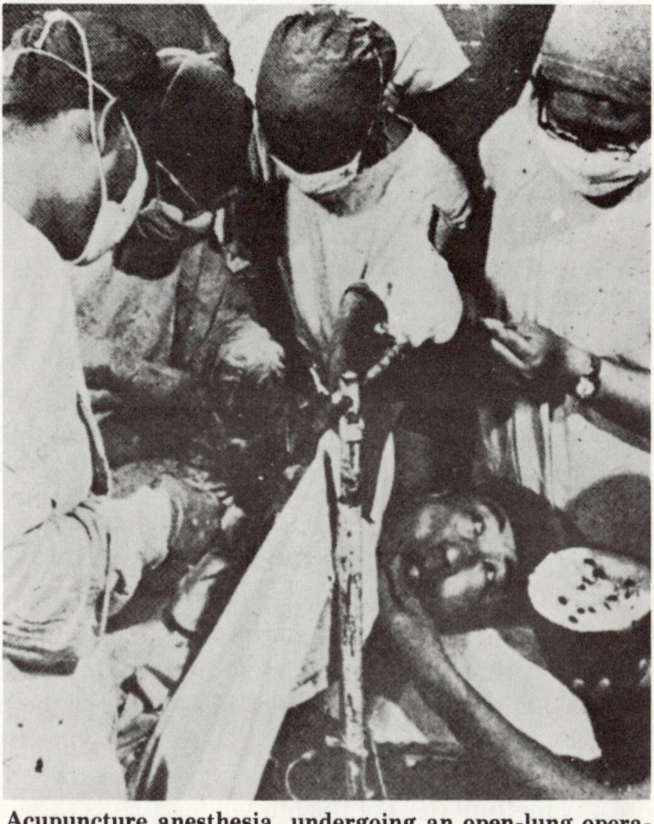

Acupuncture anesthesia, undergoing an open-lung operation at the Peking Tuberculosis Research Institute, China. *(New China News)*

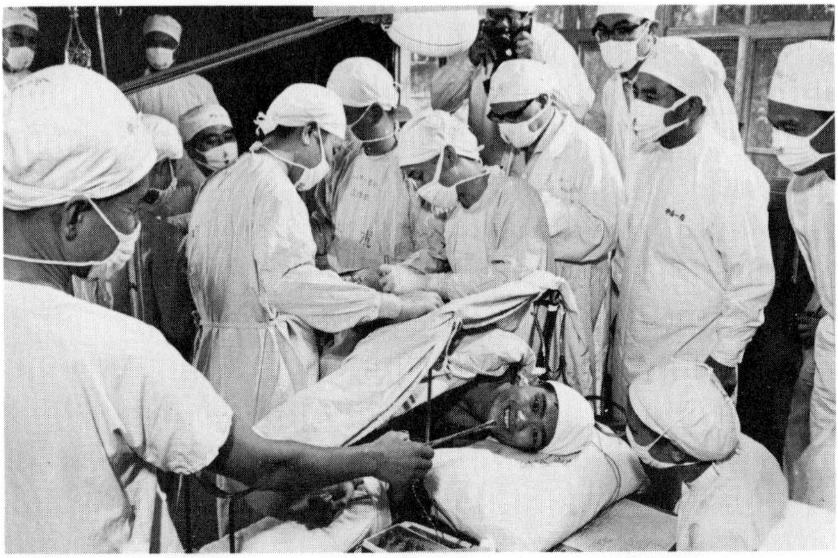

Acupuncture anesthesia—the patient smiles at the stone taken from his own kidney. The operation is surrounded by spectators. *(New China News)*

4.2 THE PRINCIPLE OF ACUPUNCTURE ANESTHESIA

Anesthetization by acupuncture involves inserting one or more needles into certain points of a patient's body. Patients are fully conscious, yet dulled to pain during operations. This effect is called analgesia, which is induced by needling certain points. The use of acupuncture anesthesia includes the accurate placement of the acupuncture needle and a knowledge of specific acupuncture points (mostly around the ear) and lines in the body with a correlation of the points that are useful in supplying analgesia and that these points must be stimulated for at least 20 to 50 minutes for sufficient anesthesia of the part of the body to be treated surgically. At the same time, needling is believed to produce a regulating power to restore any malfunctions of the human body. It is these two effects which work together to prevent and suppress pain.

Since no one has not been able to find a method to measure pain, it is difficult to make an accurate comparison between the analgesic effects on different regions produced by needling points on different parts of the body. However, the Chinese have proved through clinical practice that stimulating certain points produces effects on particular organs or regions of the body. This shows that selection of points for needling is a relatively important factor in acupuncture anesthesia.

It is clear that the whole principle is related to the nervous system as one shall see from the following:

1) The brain — central nervous center.

Electroencephalgraphy (EEG) is the study of the electrical activity of the brain. Usually the activity is recorded from electrodes placed on the scalp or beneath the cerebral cortex. Such a device is called an electroencephalogram (EEG). When an adult is relaxed, the normal EEG is from 8-13 HZ., with alpha rhythm, having an amplitude of 50 micro-volt peak-to-peak. A patient is fully conscious when acupunctural anesthetization is administered. Therefore, whatever he feels inevitably passes on to the brain which plays the primary role in the functional regulation of the body. Feeling produced by needling the points and pain sensation resulting from the operation invariably go to the brain; hence the brain is the center where the two react on each other. Experiments in China have shown that needling a normal and healthy person could produce an EEG of inhibitory effect. Such an effect differed when a different point was needled. The needling may be done by hand, or electricity; in some cases the effect is produced by injections of distilled water at certain points.* Anyhow, this is to raise the pain threshold (the minimum quantity of a stimulus needed to produce pain sensation) which is a function of time and type of stimulus. This explains why an induction period of at least twenty minutes is needed before operation. In acupuncture anesthesia, it is understood that the pain threshold is greatly elevated so the

This is to eliminate the defect resulting from the uneven manipulation of the needle by the anesthetist.

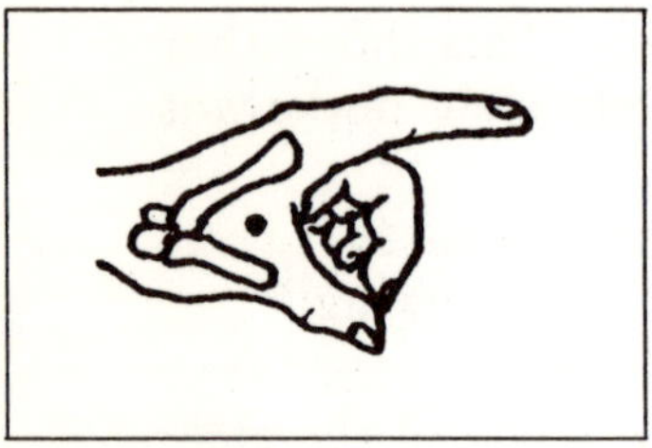

Hoku point.

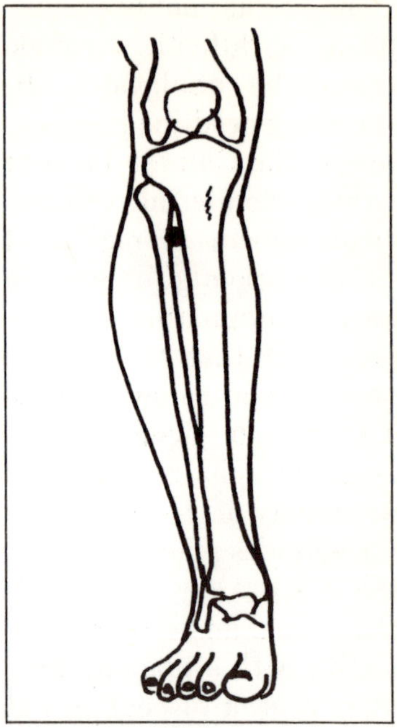

Tsuslani point.

pain stimuli produced by the incision of the skin and muscles does not register. The incision is sometimes many centimeters long, and the operation may last several hours. This produces a great deal of surgical trauma, making it a strong stimulation to the body tissue. But perception of pain is prevented by continuous manipulation of the needles throughout the operation. These two types of impulses (pain and acupuncture needling) react and counterreact with each other in the brain. Therefore, the effects of acupuncture anesthesia can be related to its action on the central nervous system.

2) The nerve fibers.

Anesthetization by acupuncture also depends on the normal functioning of nerve conduction. This is so because normal nerves are needed to carry the impulse to and from the brain. The Chinese have observed the following:

When a patient with the lower part of the body paralyzed was needled in a point (called Tsusanli) just below the knee, the patient was not responsive* to the needle. There was no change in EEG; pain threshold remained the same. But when needled the Hoku, a point between the metacarpe of the thumb and forefinger, he was responsive to the needle and the pain threshold was increased. In another case, the patient was paralyzed on one side of the body. Needling the Hoku on the paralyzed side produced nothing, while needling the healthy side would increase the pain threshold. Again, they tried it on another patient and applied regional anesthesia in his abdomen by drug. When the anesthetic was in effect, needling the Tsusanli did not cause the patient to respond to the stimulation. There was no change in pain threshold either. After the anesthetic effect disappeared, the process was repeated. The patient was then responsive to the needle; pain threshold was substantially increased. The same procedure was applied to a healthy person and to a completely paralyzed person. The results were that the acupuncture stimulation of the healthy patient was propagated fast and that of the paralyzed person was not propagated at all.

After two hours of this observation, the blood test on the healthy one revealed that glucose, red blood cells and white blood cells had been substantially increased; while that of the paralyzed showed no change at all.

All these indicate clearly that only under the normal functioning of nerve conduction can acupuncture be effectively applied.

Meanwhile, the Chinese also observed that the closer to the nerves, the acupuncture site was, the more tranquilizing the effect. In the case of the thyroid gland operation, acupuncture sites, in the past, were taken in the arm; but now they are close to the nerve endings of the

****Responsive—feelings of soreness, numbness, swelling, and heaviness.***

neck. This has produced a better result. The later means of stimulating the nerves facilitate a faster transmission of the acupuncture stimulus to the brain and spinal cord and simultaneously reduces the painful feeling due to the operation.

3) The nerve endings.

The endings of sensory nerves are the basic units used to produce analgesia by acupuncture. In order to produce the effect of acupuncture anesthesia, it is important to get the nerve endings stimulated, which causes conduction of nerve impulses and a series of reflex actions.

As we have just seen, needling the Hoku point of a healthy person could increase the pain threshold substantially. However, had the same point been first injected with conventional local anesthesia, the subject was not responsive to the acupuncture needling at all. There was also no change in pain threshold. To further understand the change of the pain threshold caused by needling certain specific point, the Chinese tried a point between the metacarpi of second and third fingers. This point does not fall on the course of a meridian and is not an acupuncture point. Surprisingly enough, the results from needling were basically the same as those of Hoku point. The subject was responsive to the needling and there was a substantial increase in the pain threshold. Meanwhile, tests were also made to measure blood contents, heart beat, blood pressure, body temperature and skin temperature. It was also found that the results of change were basically similar to each other. This is to say that nerve endings are all over and everywhere, the pain threshold will be increased provided that the nerve endings are normal and thus responsive to the needling.

Clinical practices and experiments have proved that the site for needling is not very important, so long as the stimulus reaches normal nerve endings and is transmitted,

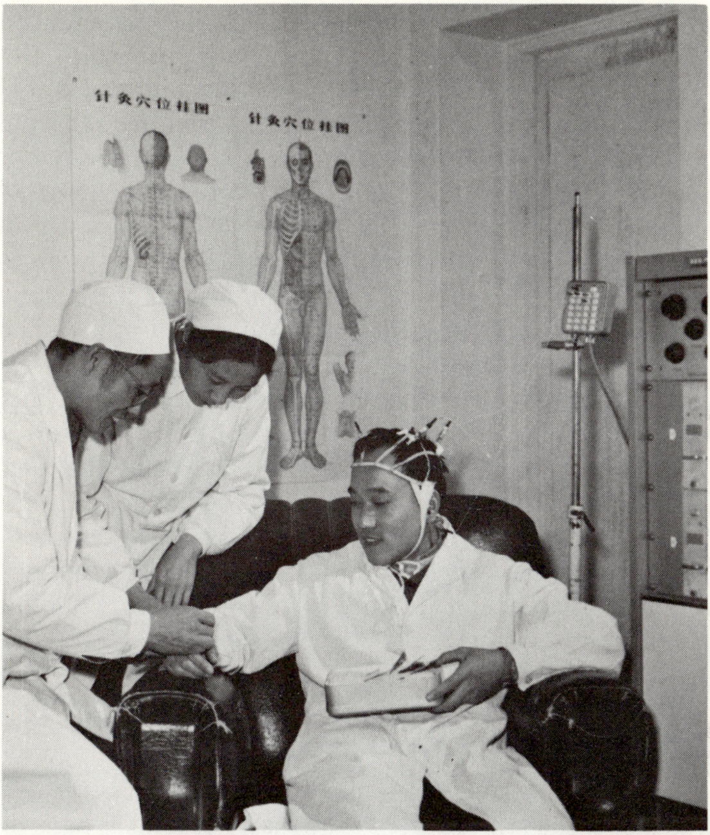

Members of a research group on the theory of acupuncture anesthesia experiment on themselves to study the effects of acupuncture on the central nervous system. *(Courtesy of the San Francisco Journal.)*

then by normal nerve conduction, to a normal central nervous system.

The site may be a conventional point, or a nerve ending or any specific point. This phenomenon can be explained in terms of bioenergetics. We learn that the cell is the basic source of all bioelectric potentials. The bioelectric potential of a cell is defined as the difference in potential existing across the cell membrane. Experimental investigations have shown that the external resting potential of a polarized cell is −90 millivolts with respect to the inside of the cell. The potential of a depolarized cell is +20 millivolts. This change in patient which results from some form of stimulation generates a travelling wave or impulse to and from the brain. Let's consider a group of cells in a particular area. The process of depolarizing all cells at the same time by stimulation is called synchronous depolarization. This may happen in an acupuncture point or a nerve ending. If the stimulation causes only one cell or a few cells to depolarize, the action of this cell depolarizing will then act as a stimulus on its adjacent cell, — thus making it depolarize, also. The process of chain reaction is called asynchronous depolarization. This may happen when needling a point around a nerve ending.

Therefore, basing on the above observation and experiments, one can conclude that the principle of acupuncture anesthesia depends mainly on the normal functioning of our nervous system.

4.3 IS ACUPUNCTURE ANESTHESIA PSYCHOSOMATIC?

It is known that a person's mental state exercises certain influence on the stimuli from the sensory organs. If he is in excellent spirits, sensitivity to stimuli may be reduced and hence the pain threshold is raised. Mental stability on the part of a patient coupled with his subjective dynamic role can bring better results to anesthetization by acupunture. Again, this can be explained in terms of bio-energetics. The change of impedance over the skin is called the exosomatic response. The appearance of a voltage is termed the endosomatic response. Both events respond to an emotional stimulus, if the subject is psychologically excited or in an elevated state. Then, they reflect a change in the activity of the autonomic nervous system. This is why Western medicine regards acupuncture anesthesia as being psychosomatic in nature. However, this can only partly explain the matter, because the patient's initiative alone cannot replace acupuncture anesthesia in carrying out an operation. It is the effect of regulation, analgesia, and the patient's initiative that constitute the stimulus to raise the patient's threshold for pain. Expressed mathematically it can be as follows:

Regulation + Analgesia + Self suggestion = Acupuncture Anesthesia.

4.4 IS ACUPUNCTURE ANESTHESIA DUE TO HYPNOSIS

The theory of meridians and the forces of Yin and Yang do not adequately explain the phenomenon of anesthesia by acupuncture. For one thing, no neurophysiological or electronic engineer in the Western world has been able to demonstrate that meridians exist.

From the pragmatic standpoint, the question arises whether it is really necessary to explain *how* it works, as long as it works. However, except for the area of religion man will always seek specific explanations of the unknown.

One theory to explain the success of acupuncture anesthesia is that it is nothing more than a refined form of hypnosis. The power of suggestion has long been recognized. Operations have been performed many times where hypnotic suggestion was the only anesthesia used.

There are several reasons why hypnosis does not explain acupuncture anesthesia. First, in observing the patient anesthetized by hypnosis and the patient anesthetized by acupuncture one may observe two entirely different expressions. The hypnotized patient usually has a characteristic drowsy, lethargic, slow motion type of appearance. The acupunctured patient is alert, clear minded, and the tone of speech is crisp as compared to the characteristic tone of the hypnotized patient. One expert in hypnosis, a psychiatrist, has postulated that the hypnotic state of acupuncture is different in that the acupunctured patient is in a state of hyper awareness rather than withdrawn from his environment as is the hypnotized patient. This does not seem logical, as the very means by which hypnosis anesthesia is accomplished is the narrowing of the patient's contact with his environment. In this way, he can concentrate on the vocal suggestions which produce anesthesia.

A second objection to the hypnosis theory is that there is no evidence that acupuncture anesthetists use the spoken word to accomplish anesthesia. If it is shown that they do not verbally suggest anesthesia to the patient, hypnosis could only result in this case from implication. To those who have witnessed the difficulty of accomplishing verbal-

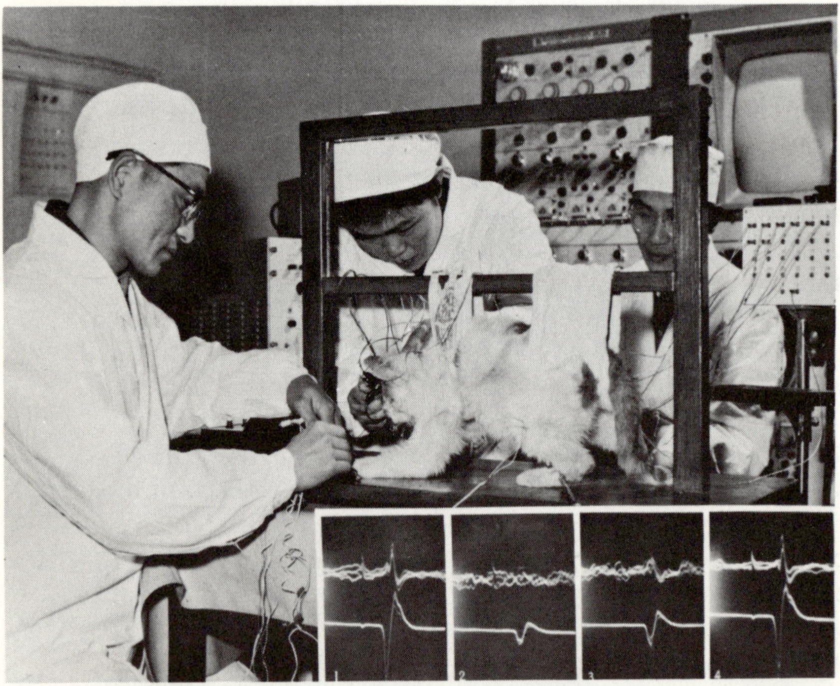

Scientists in Peking experiment on awake cat to study the analgesic effect of acupuncture. *(Courtesy of the San Francisco Journal)*

ly imposed hypnosis anesthesia, it is unreasonable to expect that a patient will develop surgical anesthesia by hinting or indirect, implied suggestion.

Authorities state that only ten to fifteen percent of the adult population is amenable to hypnosis for surgical anesthesia. Statistically, the record for acupuncture is much better than this, and also the types of operations done under acupuncture anesthesia have generally, been much bigger operations. Acupuncture patients have ranged from two-day infants to eighty-year old men, while hypnosis patients have never been younger than five years old.

Lastly, the Chinese point out that they have also successfully applied acupuncture techniques to animals both for treating diseases and anesthesia. Animals do not respond to hypnosis.

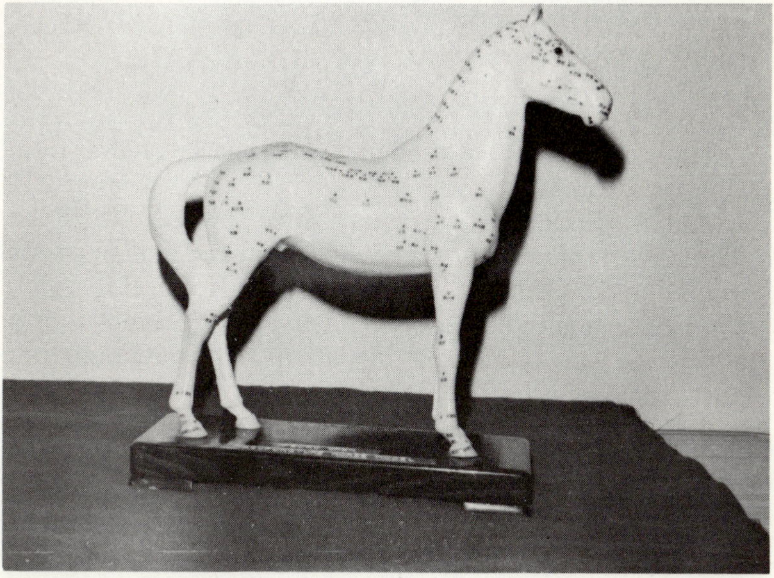

Acupuncture horse model.

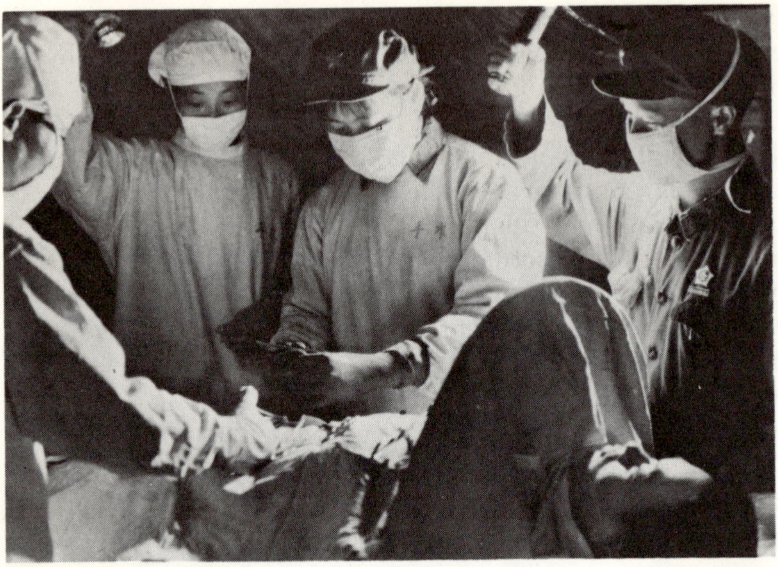

Operation under acupuncture anesthesia.

4.5 WATCHING THE OPERATIONS—CAESAREAN DELIVERY, AND REMOVAL OF A NAIL.

The following two accounts are special news from Canton, China:

"On April 19, the fourth day since the opening of the Trade Fair, there were fifty to sixty local and foreign guests invited to the Canton City First People's Hospital to watch the performances of Caesarean delivery and removal of a steel nail from thigh bone in patient, when acupuncture anesthesia was the sole anesthetic.

Delivering a baby by Caesarean operation is not something new, but the use of acupuncture as anesthesia is quite recent. The result is marvelous. The patient was a thirty-seven year old housewife. After two needles were inserted in each of her legs for sometime, the surgeons began to incise the skin and open the abdomen. The

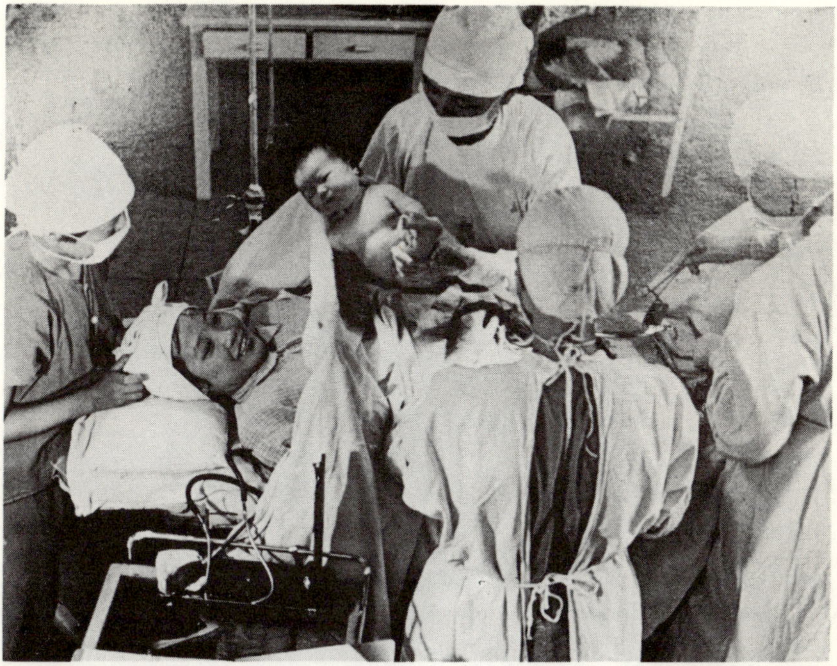

Caesarean delivery under acupuncture anesthesia.

patient was fully conscious, looked calm and pleasant. She did not feel any pain whatsoever. After a period of five minutes a baby was delivered from the mother. The baby was a boy and weighed ten pounds. The guests were all surprised by this wonderful performance, applauded and congratulated the mother. After another thirty minutes, the surgeons finished cleaning and stitching up the incision.

The operation started at 9:25 a.m. and ended at 10:00 a.m. It lasted only thirty-five minutes.

There were four surgeons, including the chief, attending at the operation. They were all female. Besides, there were two other female medical workers, one administering acupuncture anesthesia, and the other measuring the housewife's blood pressure during the operation.

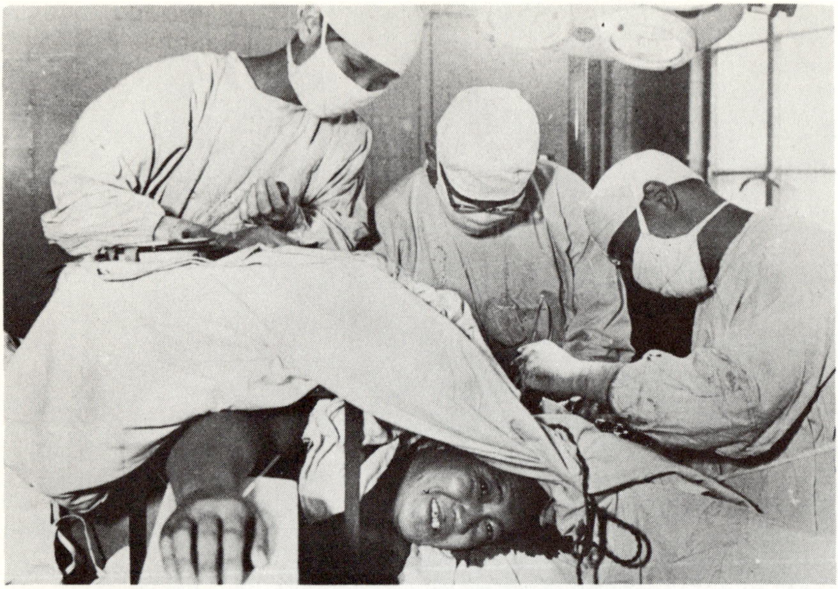

Open-brain operation under acupuncture anesthesia.

Another operation was for removal of a nail from a 44 year old lady. Three years ago, she suffered from arthritis and had a nail inserted in her left thigh bone by surgery. After her arthritis was healed, she was ready to have the nail removed. Applying the technique of acupuncture anesthesia, it only took 15 minutes to finish the whole operation."

Removal of an Inflamed Gall Bladder (China Reconstruct Oct. '71)

Under a large shadowless lamp, a 59-year old printer lays quietly on the operation table of the Third Teaching Hospital of the Peking Medical College, waiting for the doctors to remove an inflamed gall bladder which had troubled him for years.

There was no clumsy, complex anesthetic apparatus in the gleaming white operation room, and no smell of anesthetics. An anesthetist stuck four 5-cm needles slightly thicker than a human hair into points on the outside of the patient's calves and between his first and second toes. While twirling the needles in his feet, she asked "How does it feel, Old Tang?"

"A bit sore at first," he replied. "Now it's numb."

For 20 minutes the anesthetist kept twirling the four needles alternately. Then with the patient perfectly conscious, two surgeons began the operation.

While Tang felt as if a pen point had been drawn painlessly down his abdomen, a surgeon had made the incision in his abdomen wall. Examining the abdominal cavity, the surgeons found that the gall bladder had more adhesions with other organs than they had expected, and that it would take longer to cut it free than originally planned. So the anesthetist stuck a needle each into a point on the inward side of both feet to prolong the anesthetic effect.

All through the three-hour operation, the patient was calm and at ease. His blood pressure, breathing and pulse remained normal. He talked with the doctors, nurses and anesthetist and co-operated with them. The only time he felt uncomfortable was when the gall bladder was being cut, when the pull on the organ made him feel pressure on his abdomen, difficulty in breathing and bit nauseous. He had no postoperative complications and he was discharged from the hospital after a normal confinement.

ANIMAL SURGERY (Acupuncture Anesthesia Used in Animal Surgery, The San Francisco Journal, Oct. 25, '72)

Acupuncture anesthesia, an achievement scored by Chinese Medical personnel, is being successfully applied to animal surgery as well as to operations on human beings.

The Peking Municipal Veterinary Hospital and The Army Horse Disease Prevention and Treatment Center of the Peking units of the Chinese People's Liberation Army have used acupuncture anesthesia over the past two years for operations on the chest, neck, limbs and other parts of the body of 360 horses, mules, donkeys, cattle and pigs, and achieved a 95 percent success rate.

Acupuncture anesthesia induces analgesia and to a certain extent, readjusts the functioning of the organs of the ailing animals. Therefore it can deal with the acute pain and physiological disorder accompanying surgery and ensure a smooth operation.

This method is particularly effective for seriously ill animals with irregular heart beat that cannot be anesthetized. Such operations have none of the side effects caused by anesthetics and usually require only simple electric anesthetic apparatus which is easy to handle.

In October of 1970, the Peking Municipal Veterinary Hospital and the Army Horse Disease Center formed a scientific research group which improved the auricular needling anesthesia method used by other units in treating horses and mules and simplified the method by using only one needle on one acupuncture point and developed the method of electric manipulation of the needle. The group made further study and comparisons on animals and finally found more points that can induce more satisfactory analgesic effect.

One day, a 7-month pregnant mare suffering from abdomen swelling and constipation was sent to the hospital with a count of 100 heart beats per minute. Such a case would have been incurable in the past. This time, the operation went smoothly with acupuncture anesthesia. Immediately after the operation, the horse stood up to drink water and the heart-beat returned to normal. After a period of treatment, the horse fully recovered and safely delivered a colt.

4.6 PERSONAL EXPERIENCE OF A PATIENT

Acupuncture has recently been used as an anesthetic and the following story tells the experience of a young teacher from Hong Kong, Miss Kun. Miss Kun suffered from appendicitis. Her operation took place in the People's Second Hospital in Canton in mid-August 1970. The following is her narrative of this experience.

"I was at the hospital well before the operation was to take place. The hospital staff explained to us (those who were to have the acupuncture operation) different views of acupuncture anesthesia. Only those who were willing to undergo the operation would receive it. I thought it was a good idea so I said that I was willing.

After I was placed on the operation table, the staff carefully punctured two needles into my right ear. They then punctured seven needles into my right leg. At this point an electrical current was connected with the needles. I felt some vibration and a slight sensation of numbness, but I did not feel any pain. Last of all, two needles were punctured into the part of my body where the operation was to be performed; one on each side. After about ten minutes three doctors and five nurses began working on the operation. While operating, some nurses talked to me, giving me all the encouragement and reassurance I needed. One of the nurses kept a running narration of my blood pressure to the doctor. I was completely confident. I first saw the doctor use some kind of blade and then some scissors. At one time I felt a sensation of coming down in an elevator. Well before the operation I had been warned that I would have some strange sensation when an organ was disconnected. This might have been that occasion. After an hour I felt the doctor stitching me up, layer after layer. The electricity was then cut off and the needles were taken out. I was told that those who were placed under normal anesthesia would feel dizzy, suffer headaches and maybe even vomit or lose consciousness. I suffered none of these affects. Ordinarily, after an operation, the patient will throw up anything taken in, but I had porridge the first day and regular meals the second day. I think acupuncture is really safe, effective and economical."

4.7 SPECIALTIES OF ACUPUNCTURE ANESTHESIA

Acupuncture anesthesia is still a new technique. Although there are still problems and room for improvement, it has already proved to be safe, simple, easy, effective and economical. The following give a general survey of this anesthetization.

1. Convenience.

General and local anesthesia can be produced without using drugs which can produce resultant complications. The effect is not less than in any other traditional anesthetic. It is applicable regardless of equipment, climate and geographical condition.

2. Consciousness.

Patients are fully awake during operations when this kind of anesthetization is used. Apart from being dulled to pain, they are normal in other physiological functions.

3. Cooperation with the surgeon.

The surgeon can ask the patient to move the relative part of the body so as to know how the patient feels and reacts. In the meantime, the process of operation can be adjusted accordingly. Take thyroidectomy for example, the surgeon can freely talk to the patient to determine the condition of vocalization. In orthopedic operations, such as plastic surgery of the finger muscles and tendons, it makes possible the patients retaining the functions of his fingers and moving them as usual. This, coupled with the patient's active co-operation, helps the doctor find the injured muscles and tendons easily. After the operation,

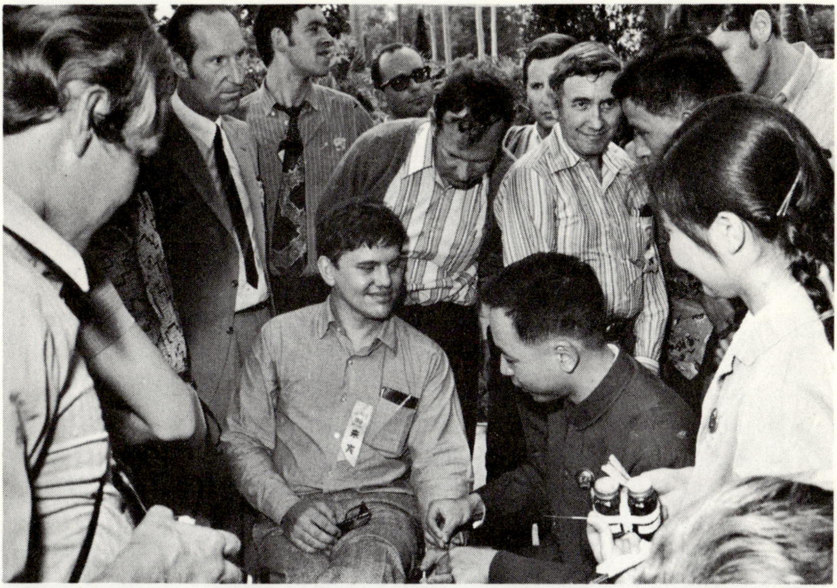

Foreign visitors to China are always anxious to experience acupuncture.

the patient can immediately move his fingers to test the results. Once there was a patient who was operated for cancer of alimentary canal. Five needles were inserted to produce anesthesia. The skin was cut, sheared through the ribs and chest cavity opened up. At this point, the patient felt as if he were pressed under a great weight, and his alimentary canal and associated organs moved from left to right as he breathed, thus hindering the operation. The surgeon asked the patient to breathe slowly and evenly with the abdomen. (A method he had practiced many times before the operation.) This breathing technique quickly reduced the feeling of pressure, and the alimentary canal and other organs settled down. The operation went on without a hitch. As soon as the patient was brought back to his ward, he was able to speak with his family. The next day he could eat and drink, and the day after was able to sit up. His strength returned quickly, and a week later he was walking around.

4. No Side Effects.

Acupuncture anesthesia helps prevent disorder in the patient's physiological functions during the operation, and, after its completion, avoid post-operative harmful effects from the use of anesthesia.

5. Normal Functions.

Needling techniques can even strengthen the patient's positive factors to resist diseases and can regulate the functions of the organism. As a result, the patient's blood pressure, pulse and breathing in general remain normal during the operation. Incisions heal and functions of the organisms concerned are restored quickly and satisfactorily after the operation. Consequently, the patient can move about and take food early. In the cases of patients who suffer from poor functionings of liver, kidneys or lungs, high blood pressure, debility from serious disease, shock or are sensitive to anesthetics, anesthetization by drugs is not advisable, while acupuncture anesthesia offers safe operations.

4.8 DISCUSSION ON CLINICAL EXPERIENCE IN ACUPUNCTURE ANESTHESIA

(Peking Hospital Worker, by Hung Yi, The San Francisco Journal July 5, 1972)

Staff members of the third hospital attached to the Peking Medical College recently held a discussion about their experience in acupuncture anesthesia and analyzed its special characteristics from various angles. Their speeches at the discussion follow:

Acupuncture Anesthesia Develops in Struggle.

by *Chow Kuan-nan* (attending physician of the surgical department):

Acupuncture anesthesia is a new anesthetizing technique. Needling is used to stimulate a certain location of the body in one or several points to make the patient feel soreness, distention, heaviness or numbness so as to induce analgesia and facilitate surgery. In 1958, our staff studied the experience of other hospitals, started to investigate acupuncture anesthesia. We undertook clinical practice and performed more than 30 operations under acupuncture anesthesia. But this project was interrupted by revisionists spreading such fallacies as "Chinese traditional medicine is not scientific" and "acupuncture anesthesia has no practical value."

During the Great Proletarian Cultural Revolution, our testing of acupuncture anesthesia resumed under the guidance of Chairman Mao's revolutionary line. Under the leadership of the hospital revolutionary committee, there was formed a special group of patients and treatment wards set aside for this purpose. As a result, acupuncture anesthesia has made rapid progress in our hospital. There have been performed 1,200 operations under acupuncture anesthesia in 1970 and 1971.

Acupuncture anesthesia has developed from only body needle placement to many other methods including auricular needling and the combination of auricular needling and insertion of needles into points of the body. The scope of application has been widened from a few simple minor operations to a variety of operations, including removal of the gall-bladder, uterus, cancer of the esophagus and part of the stomach, and operations on the limbs.

Characteristic Features of Acupuncture Anesthesia
by *Lio Chao* (anesthetist):

In my experience acupuncture anesthesia does not need complicated apparatus. It is safe, simple, easy to master and costs practically nothing. Its application interferes very little with an operation and patient regains his health quickly.

For patients with poor liver, kidney, heart or lung

function, high blood pressure, or who are in a critical state or are oversensitive to anesthetics, acupuncture anesthesia is safer than administering anesthetics.

A patient suffering from an extra-uterine pregnancy was sent to our hospital. Excessive bleeding led to hemorrhagic shock. The pulse was weak and she was nonresponsible to external stimuli. A patient in such a condition is a poor anesthesia risk. Distention of the abdomen, or pneumonia were some of the complications expected. Acupuncture anesthesia was used. Needles were inserted into acupuncture points and within five minutes her blood pressure rose. During the operation the patient felt all right, except when blood clots were manually removed from the abdomen. The operation was uneventful. The patient could take solid food the next day. There were no complications and the patient was discharged from the hospital after a short recovery.

Li Feng-ming (opthalmologist):

Acupuncture anesthesia has proved effective in eye operations. It helps avoid edema of the tissues in the zone operated on. This is helpful in making an accurate incision on the conjunctiva. Post-operative side-effects are slight and the patient recovers quickly. When anesthetic is administered for an operation to correct squinting, success or failure is known only after the effects of the drug wear off. But when anesthetization is done by acupuncture, the patient's eyeballs can move freely and the doctor can ascertain the result of the operation then and there.

Chang Li-chu (a doctor in the gynecology and obstetrics department)

I have been a teacher and doctor for over 20 years. I have performed various kinds of gynecological and obstetric operations. Yet I was skeptical about using acupuncture needles to induce analgesia.

I performed an operation under acupuncture anesthesia for the first time in 1970. At that time, acupuncture anesthesia was already popular in our hospital, but I was doubtful of its success. I was assigned an operation to tie up the oviducts. I prepared a local anesthetic so that if acupuncture anesthesia failed, I could use it. However, the anesthesia provided by acupuncture was highly successful and the patient felt no pain during the operation. This gave me greater confidence and the doctors of our department now have applied the method in Caesarean section, removal of ovarian tumors, uterectomy and other operations. All were successful.

Li Mei-chih (obstetrician-gynecologist):

When general anesthetic is used, the patient is completely passive during the operation. But when acupuncture anesthesia is used, surgeon, anesthetist and patient can work in close coordination. The surgeon acquaints the patient with the nature and course of the operation in advance to gain the patient's cooperation. Gynecological operations require that the patient relax the muscles of the abdominal wall and breathe evenly. Surgeons must pay more attention to the state of the patient than when general anesthetics are used. Therefore acupuncture anesthesia places stricter demands on the medical workers, higher skill and a strong will to serve the people heart and soul. The operation must be performed with precision, steadiness, care and speed. Before the operation begins, the length and location of the incision is set. Through pre-operation examinations must be done if you want to avoid unnecessary probing on the table and achieve good results.

Chang Li-chu,

I have been to the countryside making rounds on a number of occasions. When we performed major operations, we had to call an ambulance from our hospital to bring us the necessary apparatus and anesthetics. There were many unexpected mishaps, and treatment would be delayed. I feel keenly that the countryside badly needs a simple method of anesthesia. Popularization of acupuncture anesthesia is of significance in carrying out Chairman Mao's instruction "in medical and health work, put the stress on the rural areas."

Wang Su-chen (head nurse):

Patients under acupuncture anesthesia are easier to provide nursing care. After the operation, they don't suffer from the side effects common after the administering of general or spinal anesthetics. An appendectomy under spinal anesthesia often gives the post-operative patient headaches, dizziness, abdominal distention and even retention of urine. It is even more difficult to nurse patients after operations with general anesthesia. Patients after operation with acupuncture anesthesia can take food and move about earlier and recuperate faster.

Wang Kuan (doctor in charge of acupuncture anesthesia):

Acupuncture anesthesia is a brilliant example of the combination of Chinese traditional and Western medicines, and has many special features. But like other new things, it has raised some problems that still have to be solved. For instance, at certain stages in some operations, patients still feel some pain, and at some certain points the pain is still high; some patients feel uncomfortable when the internal organs are manipulated; and in some abdominal operations, the patient's abdominal operations, the patient's abdominal muscles are not satisfactorily relaxed, and this creates difficulties for the operator.

Ma Li-hua (acupuncture anesthesia doctor):

Acupuncture anesthesia is used in operations on all parts of the body in various parts of China, but in our experience it has not been successful for all operations. In some difficult operations with serious adhesion of intro-abdominal organs that call for extensive exploration, acupuncture anesthesia does not work well. But we are confident that these difficulties will be overcome.

Chou Kuan-han:

On the question of why acupuncture has an anesthetic effect, medical workers in various parts of the country have conducted research and opinions and explanations vary. This question still remains to be solved.

Chapter 5

Is the Meridian System the same as the Nervous System ?

Is the Meridian System the same as the Nervous System ?

The principle of acupuncture anesthesia depends mainly on the normal functioning of our nervous system, one may wonder whether the meridian system is the same as the nervous system. This is a rather controversial question. The reader may be able to find the answer after reading the following presentation.

5.1 SIMILARITY IN NATURE

First, a comparative analysis of the results of acupuncture anesthesia and segmental innervation find that meridians and nerves in a large measure correspond with each other. The pathway which connects different parts of the body surface and certain internal organs is called meridian. The meridian links up all the viscera and different parts of the body surface, making the human body an integrated whole. Modern physiology has also verified that different parts of the body are interconnected. However, physiologists maintain that connections are mainly affected through the nerves. In conclusion, the Chinese consider that the meridian includes not only the nerves and blood vessels but may include certain other connecting pathways and activities inside the human body. The laws governing them are still unknown. Neurology defines a nerve as consisting of nerve fibers, together with their blood vessels and lymphatic vessels and fiber coverings. Comparison makes it clear both these two systems possess the properties of irritability (the ability to respond to a stimulus), conductivity (the ability to conduct nerve impulses), and integration (the ability to organize and regulate impulses).

Another indication of the close similarity of the meridian system and the nervous system is the close location of some three hundred acupuncture points to nerve fibers. Half of them lie direct above nerve fibers and the other half are no further than 1/2 centimeter away from nerve fibers.

However there are some theories which can be explained by the meridians which cannot be explained in terms of neuroanatomy and neurophysiology. For instance, according to the meridian theory, the kuangming point in the lower part of the leg is the main point for treating eye diseases. Good results have been obtained by needling this point to induce analgesia for eye operations. But how does needling this point affect the eyes and how are these two parts connected? It is very difficult to explain these facts with our present knowledge of neurology. The pain that is produced with thermal stimulation of certain parts of the limbs, sensitivity to pain appears in the corresponding areas on the ears. This shows that points on the ears have certain specific connections with other parts of the body. Each of the twelve meridians runs in pairs, one to each side of the body. If one side is stimulated, the other side is also affected. Explaining these connections with our present knowledge of neurology is also difficult. One explanation is that the study of neurology has been limited and incomplete, and the functions of the various systems in the human body are very complex and delicate.

One of the medical doctors mentioned in the preface of this book suggests a theory based on some very fundamental neurophysiological facts. He proposes this theory in order to rebut the spontaneous skepticism of acupuncture anesthesia he has encountered in many of his medical colleagues. He does not propose that the theory does explain how acupuncture anesthesia is produced but that it could explain acupuncture anesthesia in a way that would be acceptable to Western medicine. The theory follows:

There is a fundamental neurological function known as the spinal reflex arc. This phenomenon is familiar to all of us as the knee jerk reflex which a physician normally produces by tapping the tendon below the knee with a little rubber hammer.

What happens when the tendon is tapped is that the leg jerks forward. The nerve signal for this is very simple. The stimulus goes up the sensory nerve in the tendon into the spinal cord, makes a few connections and then goes to the muscles that make the leg jerk forward.

The brain is not needed for this to occur. The spinal cord could be completely severed any place above the level of the nerves involved in this reflex. The above reflex would still occur.

However, physicians know that the brain does exert some control over this reflex. Thus, if the spinal cord connection between the lower spine and the brain is cut, the knee jerk is much greater, in other words a controlling factor has been eliminated.

Therefore, even a simple spinal reflex arc stimulus is transmitted upperward to the brain and from the brain certain other signals are sent. The latter signals do not necessarily have to go back to the leg. They can go to other parts of the body. For instance if the stimulus to the tendon below the knee is severe enough to cause what is called neurogenic shock, signals from the brain go to blood vessels in all parts of the body to produce this condition of shock.

In simplest terms, the doctor's theory is that acupuncture anesthesia is produced by interruption of reflexes and nerve pathways that conduct pain. The stimulus of the needle goes to the spinal cord. There it makes connections with nerves which go to the brain. Nerves from the brain carry another signal to a certain specific organs. Why stimulation of certain acupuncture points results in anesthesia of a particular location is not explainable at this time but the pathways are.

5.2 PHILOSOPHY vs SCIENCE — BACKGROUND AND COMPARISON

Let us not forget that the Chinese meridians were described in ancient Chinese medical treatises longer than two thousand years ago. Two specific ideas can be explored. This means two things.

1. The descriptions of the meridians and their concepts have not been developed. It is true, however, that while historical discoveries in Chinese medicine have been colossal, there had been in recent times little progress in the development of the original discoveries.* In other words, the ancient descriptions, though some of them seem accurate, might not be complete or even correct in the scientific sense. The early Chinese hardly bothered to develop more than an elementary knowledge of bones, nerves, blood vessels, etc. This does not mean that they did not know of their existance, but the emphasis of their study was on how the body related to its environment, and how the organs related to one another in the body. Chinese

Chen, C. Y. "History of Chinese Medical Science," Chinese Medical Institute, Hong Kong, 1969, p. 17.

people often have a tendency to initiate a new subject and then leave it for others to study. Gun power is a good example. The Chinese are ones who first invented it, but who has developed it into TNT or A bomb or H bomb. Another example is the abacus, which now in its modern form is a computer. There are many many others such as the compass, paper, brush, printing, to name just a few. Therefore, the original pattern of the meridian system may be in a scientific sense the nervous system as it was originally described. The only way we can find it out is by further investigation. One must thank and respect our wise ancestors who have passed down to us a rich treasure of findings, though some of them might not be scientific and complete.

The teachings of the Chinese forefathers have been given us to supply the needed scientific confirmation and correlation of the theories proposed by them.

2. These medical treatises were written at the time when philosophy was booming, with the Yin and Yang doctrine prevailing. Since these medical people were also philosophers, it was natural and inevitable for them to apply philosophical terms to medical theories. It is especially true when they knew it worked, but did not know how it worked. Perhaps, they had never been exposed to modern medical theories. Today, we will find them very similar to each other, if we compare terms of these two systems as indicated in the following table:

PHILOSOPHICAL TERMS	SCIENTIFIC TERMS
1. The meridian system.	A nervous system.
2. Meridians.	Nerve pathways.
3. Acupuncture points.	Sensory nerve endings.
4. Yin and Yang.	Potentials caused by positive and negative ions.
5. The five elements: Metal, water, wood, fire, and earth.	Different kinds of Stimuli and impulses.
6. Qi (life energy) — energy circulating the meridian system.	Wave of electrical depolarization along the nerve.
7. Cycles of the five elements.	Functions of the two divisions (sympathetic and parasympathetic) of the autonomic nervous system.
a. Creation cycle.	Excitation by harmones of adrenaline and norepinephrine.
b. Control cycle.	Inhibition by hormone of acetylcholine.
c. Threatening cycle.	Induction by adrenocortical hormones.

5.3 SOME BIOLOGICAL PHENOMENA ABOUT OUR BODY

There are also some laws of acupuncture which can be explained in terms of bio-energetics. For instance, according to tradition, the choice of points to be used for treatment varies with different seasons. Once one learns that the conducting properties of the body (e.g. impedance change) have been found to vary also with seasons, we then realize that this phenomenon may be related to it.

Impedance method is a technique involving the detection of an impedance change between two electrodes over a subject. This method can be applied to measure many physiological events, because the change of impedance reflects the secretion of the hormones or the functioning of the autonomic nervous system. A decrease in the subject's impedance indicates excitement. Relaxation is indicated by an increase in impedance. However, it is regretted that there has been no attempt to interpret the value of the impedance method in true physiological terms.

The routes of meridians can be traced in the body. The location is found by measuring the impedance change over the skin, because it is said that meridians have the property of less electrical impedance. However, the most familiar example of biological impedance change is that which accompanies the physiological activity of a nerve. Cole and Curtis (1939) showed that, as an impulse travels along a nerve fiber, the membrane exhibits a transient decrease in impedance.* Can it be that the property of a meridian is actually that of a nerve? The transient changes that occur in nerves can be measured and these changes can be measured in the meridian system. It is possible that the meridian system can only be found in the living body and that to identify it in a corpse is impossible because the meridian system is similar to a reflex arc or functionery nerves. This would propose that the meridian may share a

Geddes and Baker, Principles of Applied Bio-medical Instrumentation, John Wiley and Sons, Inc., New York, London, Sydney, p. 192.

pathway in the peripheral body that can not be dissected.

In summary, one may conclude that the function of a meridian is similar as that of a nerve. To make a further assumption, it may be said that a meridian may be a nerve.

5.4 THE FOURTH SYSTEM DOES NOT EXIST.

In 1962, Dr. Bonghan Kim of North Korea claimed to have discovered little groups of oval cells at acupuncture points which are connected to one another by ducts. Dr. Kim calls this a fourth system*, or Kyungrak system, the route of which is said to coincide with that of the Chinese meridians. This new system has not been reproduced or verified by any other scientist, despite intensive research, the mystery of what is called the meridian system still remains a mystery. The nervous system can be explained and related to but the meridian system has not been correlated to any known system in Western medicine.

****The other three systems are nervous, vascular and lymphatic.***

Chapter 6

Questions that are most often asked

Questions that are most often asked

Is acupuncture infallible?

According to Dr. S.W. Wu, a noted acupuncture authority from Hong Kong, "Acupuncture is beautiful, it can cure everything." In her statistics, about 70 to 80% of her patients have been effectively treated. (See my first edition entitled, "Acupuncture, Electro-acupuncture, Anesthesia.") It has also been known that acupuncture can sometimes mysteriously heal some strange ills, which may be considered incurable, or without having knowledge of its origin or cause.

Dr. Felix Mann, President of the Medical Acupuncture Society in England, says in his book, "Acupuncture — cure of many diseases," that acupuncture is good for those diseases influenced by a physiological process, e.g. duodenal ulcer, acne vulgaris, migraine; it is ineffective for those purely anatomical and uninfluencable by a physiological process, e.g. kidney stone, advanced osteoarthritis, a fully formed cataract.

Being a Western trained doctor and an acupuncturist in China, Chu Lien, in her book of "Modern Acupuncture" says that acupuncture is not infallible. Although in clinical practice, acupuncture therapy may do better than drugs for some cases, it does not mean we have to give up our present medicine and other scientific therapies. One should apply whatever therapy or a combination which can do best to the patient.

How does a patient respond to the treatment of acupuncture?

There is no definite answer. It varies with different kinds of diseases and patients. However, if the case is newly acquired, the patient can be responsive on even his first visit. If it is a serious case, it may take up to three treatments in order to see a response.

How often does the patient receive the treatment?

Usually once a day or every other day. But it is advisable to consult with the doctor for the final word.

Can everybody take the treatment of acupuncture?

No, the patient should stay away from acupuncture if under the following conditions.

1) He is too hungry, or full, or drunk, or tired, or nervous.

2) He is too weak and has serious heart attack problem.

3) It is always wise for pregnant women to avoid acupuncture treatment.

4) Try not to needle those parts that have a scar.

5) Avoid moxibustion if the patient has high blood pressure.

Are there any side effects or complications from acupuncture?

With long needles, in some areas, there is risk of organ or blood vessel penetration. Unsterile needles present a risk of infections. However, there is no other known side effects such as addicting, toxia, adverse effects.

What is the attitude in the United States towards acupuncture?

There is no definite law for or against unlicensed practitioner of acupuncture. However, to practice medicine, one has to be a licensed M.D. or D.O. There are still no official acupuncture societies. But ever since acupuncture became more widely known in the newspapers and magazines, many people have become very inquisitive about it. In general, these people can be divided into three groups:

1. The general public. The response is favorable. Many of them have tried to acquire more information by buying acupuncture literature and by attending lectures and demonstrations.

2. The "incurable" patient. For these patients, acupuncture seems to be the last possible cure for their illness. They have been treated by Western medicine, but in vain. When they hear about acupuncture, some of them try to look for an acupuncture practitioner in Chinatown, or they attempt to go to Hong Kong or China.

3. The medical profession. Some of them still remain skeptical, while some begin to be interested in investigating the technique. Both Dr. Paul D. White (Physician of the late President Eisenhower) and Dr. Walter Tkach (President Nixon's physician) have announced to send a team of doctors to China for the study of acupuncture. Dr. Wesley Hall, President of American Medical Association, has proposed to invite a team of Chinese surgeons to demonstrate the technique of acupuncture anesthesia.

Many individual medical persons are also applying to China to learn the method. Due to lack of facility, China has turned down most requests. Many just go to Hong Kong in the hope of getting to China.

What is the present world situation of acupuncture?

China, Japan, Korea, Russia, and to a lesser extent, France all have active research programs on acupuncture and naturally recognize it as a definite therapeutic system.

Acupuncture is recognized and respected throughout the Far East and has been the main medical system for over 400 million people.

Peru has recently accepted acupuncture in its own right. Austria, Italy, England, France and Germany have well-established societies of acupuncture practitioners, with headquarters in Paris.

Australia, New Zealand and South Africa have no official policy towards acupuncture and it may be practiced without interference.

In Canada and the United States, acupuncture is not a recognized medical practice. However, a corresponding school named North American College of Acupuncture in Vancouver, Canada has been established in 1971.

What is electro-acupuncture?

It is a new technique of acupuncture, by using some electronic devices to take over the manual manipulation of the needle. The traditional acupuncture gives mechanical stimulation, by hand: while the electro-acupuncture gives electrical stimulation by passing current through the needle into the patient.

What is the difference between conventional electro-therapy and electro-acupuncture?

The two operate on completely different principles. In conventional electro-therapy, it uses surface stimulation or the penetrating heating action of electromagnetic waves; while in electro-acupuncture, the needle penetrates into particular human structure and the electric current is utilized as a stimulator.

Who can learn acupuncture?

Anybody who has the desire can learn acupuncture. There isn't anything that we cannot learn. Where there is a will, there is a way.

How long does it take to learn acupuncture?

It varies with the individual. If you have extensive background of medical knowledge, then the time required to learn is, of course, much shorter. The North American College of Acupuncture in Canada, offers a corresponding course in acupuncture. Under normal study speed and promotion, the Canadian course only takes a little more than a year. It includes basic anatomy and physiology, acupuncture points and techniques and clinical practice. If you are also interested in the Chinese medical philosophy and principles of diagnosis, it takes another year. You can even go further to learn the Chinese herbiology (prescription and preparation) which requires about two years.

Where can one learn acupuncture anesthesia?

This is a new technique originated in China; therefore, China is the only place that you can learn this method of anesthesia. Many other countries have started investigating this new medical science. As of June, 1972, few operations have been successfully performed using acupuncture anesthesia; tonsillectomy in Vienna, Austria, and Louis A. Weiss Memorial Hospital, Chicago, U.S.A., skin graft in Albert Einstein College of Medicine of Yeshiva University, New York, U.S.A., and minor plastic procedures in France.

Chapter 7

Acupuncture in America

Acupuncture in America

7.1 DEVELOPMENT

Acupuncture and other methods of Chinese medicine had been generally ignored in the United States. However, this system of Chinese healing had its first contact with Americans back in 1949 when the translation of "The Yellow Emperor's Classic of Internal Medicine," in which all the basic acupuncture technique was recorded, was published. The work is credited to Ilza Veith, Ph.D., professor of medical history, who took up this great project for her doctorate thesis. Unfortunately, because of China and America participating in the Korean war in 1950, America and China had no cultural exchange and literature was not studied.

After about 22 years of little communication, the two nations are now beginning to get closer. Speaking on acupuncture alone, the first news brought back to America was by two American biologists in May 1971. They are Dr. Arthur W. Galston, professor of biology at Yale University, and Dr. Ethan Signer, associate professor of biology at Massachusetts Institute of Technology. They are believed to be the first American scientists to visit China and tour research centers since the goodwill arose between the two nations. During their two-week visit, they witnessed four operations by acupuncture anesthesia, including removal of tumor and ovary cyst. Both of them were convinced of the effectiveness of the remarkable procedure and stressed that China has undergone a lot of scientific developments of which America is not generally aware..

Since then, acupuncture has become an increasing interest in the news media and the general public. However, the medical profession still remained skeptical because these reports were not from the medical professional. In September, four American prominent physicians and their wives were invited to China by the Chinese Medical Association. They are Dr. E. Grey Dimond of Missouri Medical School, Dr. Samuel Rosen of Mount Sinai Medical School, Dr. Victor Sidel of New York's Montefiore, and Dr. Paul White of Harvard University. Since their return to America, there has been an unprecedented interest in acupuncture in the whole nation. They brought back the film of Acupuncture Anesthesia in which seven operations performed under acupuncture anesthesia were witnessed with their presence.

President Nixon's trip to China in February 1972 has helped bring acupuncture to the attention of the general public as well as medical profession. Dr. Walter R. Trach, personal physician to President Nixon, said that acupuncture anesthesia is superior to conventional anesthesia.

In Oct. the first delegation of Chinese doctors arrived in

America for a three-week visit for medical exchange.

A journal entitled "American Journal of Chinese Medicine" will make its appearance early 1973. It is expected to investigate all aspects of Chinese medicine.

In short, the period of acupuncture development is brief in America, but the enthusiastic response is excellent.

7.2 SYMPOSIA AND ORGANIZATIONS

Ever since acupuncture became a hot subject in America, there have been a lot of symposia, seminars, lectures, and gatherings of similar natures. Because acupuncture is such a new medical art in the United States, it is indeed difficult to find a knowledgeable practicing acupuncturist who can speak English and understand Western medicine.

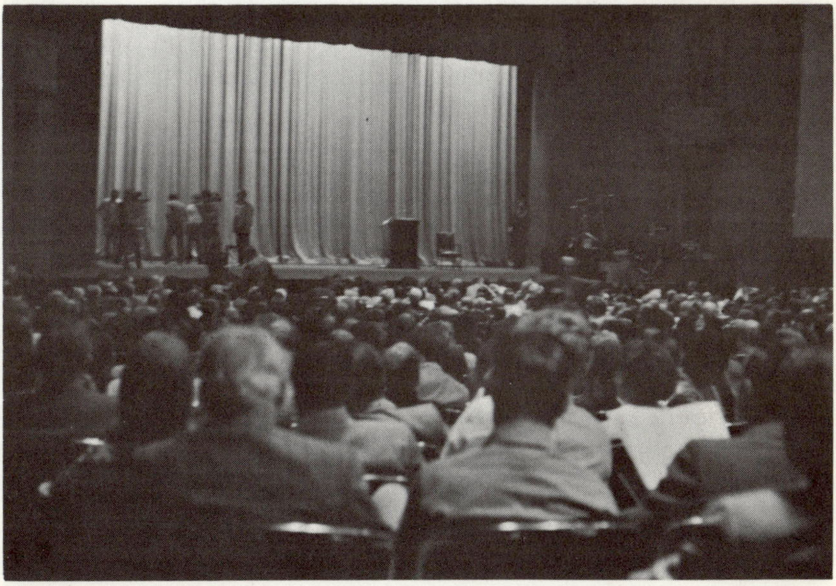

Acupuncture symposium at Stanford University, sponsored by the Academy of Parapsychology and Medicine.

The Academy of Parapsychology and Medicine has been very active in carrying out the message of acupuncture. The most successful symposium was held at Stanford University. Interest in this subject is confirmed in that an audience of 1,400 physicians and members of the allied medical community attended. It was a one-day program and the panel included:

James L. Rhee, M.D., President of the California Society of Anesthesiologists and Clinical Associate in Anesthesiology at the University of California Medical Center.

William A. McGarey, M.D., Conductor of acupuncture workshops in Arizona.

Felix Mann, M.B., B. Chir., LMCC, Founder of the Medical Acupuncture Society of Great Britain and author of five acupuncture texts on acupuncture.

C. Norman Shealy, M.D., Director of the Pain Rehabilitation Center, La Crosse, Wisconsin.

William A. Tiller, Ph.D., Professor of Stanford University.

Leonard A. Worthington, A.B., LL.B., J.D., Northern California Chairman of the Committee on Discovery Proceedings in State Bar Matters.

Frank Z. Warren, M.D., Executive Director of the National Research Society for Acupuncture.

Paul D. White, M.D., Personal physician to President Eisenhower, and one of the four doctors who visited China last September.

A more expensive seminar was sponsored by the International Hospital Supply Corporation in Hawaii. This "medical experience" cost $495 per doctor. Of course, this price also included transportation and accommodation. This symposium hosted two outstanding American physicians of Chinese ancestry and training. They are Pang Ling Man, M.D. and Calvin H. Chen, M.D., from Northville, Michigan.

Beside just talk and demonstration, concerned medical professionals and scientists also united together to form some acupuncture centers. In the East, the American Society of Chinese Medicine, Inc., was founded in early 1972 in Connecticut. In the Heart of America, there is the Acupuncture Society of America, Inc., in Kansas City. The West is not behind. The National Acupuncture Association and Acupuncture Research Institute were also formed in California.

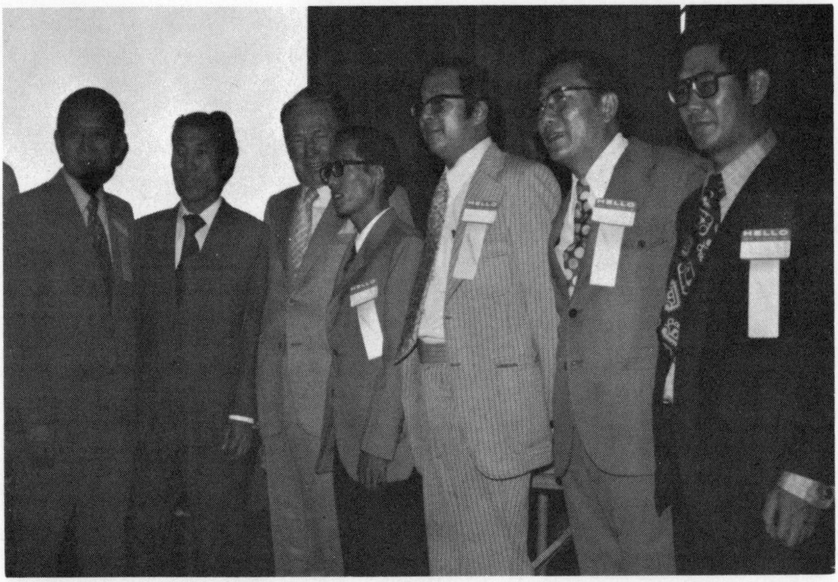

Acupuncture talk at Los Angeles City Hall. From left to right: Dr. J. Chen, Dr. Y. Choi, Mayor S. Yorty, Dr. W. Wong, Dr. J. Wong, Dr. P. Hwang, and the author, P. Chan.

7.3 THEORIES OF ACUPUNCTURE ANESTHESIA

When asked about the mechanism behind acupuncture, the Chinese offered no explanation or said that they came out with so many opinions that they are still working in this respect. In America, the most popular explanation is the spinal-gate theory proposed in 1965 by Drs. Ronald Melzack of McGill University and Patrick Wall of University College, London. This theory was originally proposed for pain pathways, not for acupuncture. It explains that there are two kinds of nerve fibers: the large alpha fibers and small fibers. The needle stimulates the first ones and thus closes a hypothetical gate in the spinal cord. This would then block nerve impulses going along the small nerve fibers to the spinal cord into the brain. Thus, the patient does not feel pain and yet he is conscious of all other sensations.

The spinal-gate theory is good only for those parts of the body below the neck; it does not explain why the needle inserted in and the hand and foot would induce analgesia for dental operations.

Recently, Drs. Man and Chen have proposed their neurological double-gate theory. According to them, there may be another "master" gate in the thalamus of the midbrain which can also accept impulses from the rest of the body. Once the gates are saturated with needling stimulation, the pain caused by surgery can not pass to the brain through the small nerve fibers (c-fibers). Their theory had been coupled and verified with findings from their clinical studies.

On February 15, 1972, Dr. H.C. Tien of Michigan Institute of Psychosynthesis also advanced the neurogenic interference theory of acupuncture anesthesia. This explains needling the hand could induce bilateral anesthesia for tonsilectomy or dental operation through intercortical pathways.

There was such a saying that the Chinese offers the American some empirical art and the American provides it with a theory.

7.4 PRESENT STATUS

Early in 1972, the U.S. Food and Drug Administration from the Department of Health, Education and Welfare placed an embargo on the import of acupuncture needles.

New York seems to be the first state to sense and to lose a taste of acupuncture. For in July, 1972, an acupuncture center was open — for only two weeks. It was run by an American internist who hired three Chinese acupuncturists in the clinic. Despite an overwhelming interest and business the state declared it unconstitutional and closed it down because those acupuncturists were practicing medicine without a license. The State Board for Medicine later ruled that acupuncture was not an accepted medical procedure at that time. That acupuncture clinic then moved to Washington, D.C.

On June 29, 1972, California Medical Association sponsored a bill (Bill #AB 1500, amended version) to permit non-licensed medical personnel to do acupuncture and other related Chinese medicine research in an approved California medical school under the supervision of a licensed physician. On August 14, 1972, Governor Reagan signed the bill.

Later in November, the House of the California Assembly on a 65-0 vote, approved another acupuncture bill (#AB 975) which would allow unlicensed persons to practice acupuncture if supervised by a licensed M.D. or dentist. The bill was also approved by the senate but vetoed by Governor Reagan with the following comment: "The research effort at medical schools is now under way. Until further research has been completed, a broadening of authority to practice acupuncture is premature. The State Board of Medical Examiners has requested that the bill be vetoed. I concur in their opposition at this time."

In an issue about acupuncture on June 2, 1972, the American Society of Anesthesiologists warns the risk and hazard of premature use of acupuncture in the United States. It admits of its potentially valuable technique, but it takes prolonged and serious study. Meanwhile, it has established its own task force to coordinate all activities concerned with acupuncture and placed its resources and expertise at the disposal of the Federal Government in pursuing acupuncture studies.

While The American Medical Association is still hesitating whether acupuncture should be included as a subject for discussion at next year's convention, it has already invited the Chinese delegation of medical profession to America for a three-week visit. More contacts between the two countries are also being planned.

Three units of National Institutes of Health have been directed to investigate acupuncture — the National Institute of General Medical Sciences, the National Institute of Neurological Diseases and Stroke, and the Fogarty International Center. On August 1, 1972, they approved to expand research programs on acupuncture for anesthesia as well as pain relief. Grants will be offered to those applicants to conduct acupuncture research. As of November, eight research units had submitted their applications.

7.5 CASE HISTORIES

Despite the uncertain status of acupuncture, the craze for acupuncture treatment, either by an M.D. or an unlicensed acupuncturist, has spread out the whole country. Among those people who claimed to be benefited by acupuncture are famous athletes like:
Roman Gabriel, Frank Leahy, Ed Lothamer, Sam McDowell, Willie McCovey, Bill Sudakis.
Singers like: Anna Moffo.
Movie stars like: Zsa Zsa Gabor, Lorne Greene.
T.V. stars like: Merv Griffin,
and even the President of California Medical Association, Dr. Thomas Elmendorf.

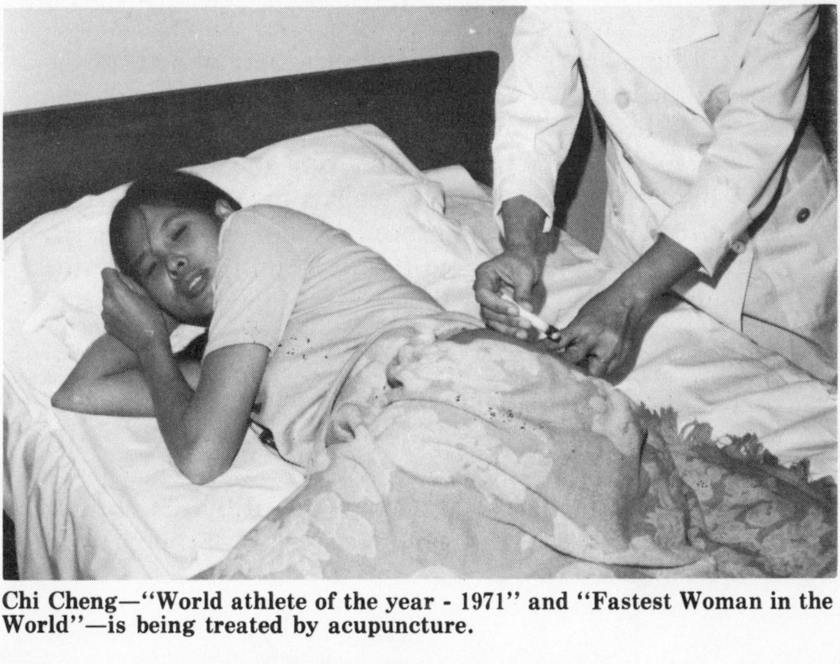

Chi Cheng—"World athlete of the year - 1971" and "Fastest Woman in the World"—is being treated by acupuncture.

The following are two reports on acupuncture, one is treatment of headache, the other is anesthesia of removal of tonsil.

Case 1: Headache

The patient is 59 years old, retired. He had suffered from severe headaches for over 25 years. He had exhausted all avenues of relief through the medical profession and eye doctors. Numerous chiropractic adjustments had not helped any. For over a year these headaches had been occurring daily from which the only relief he could get was from powerful pain relieving drugs the doctor had prescribed for him.

Since the needle treatment, (a total of four treatments, once every other day) he has been free of these headaches and is able to use his eyes to read once again.

Case 2: Tonsillectomy

This operation took place in South Bay Community Hospital, Redondo Beach, California on August 25, 1972. The patient was a 20-year old girl. Dr. Wayne Ho performed the surgery and Dr. James Chen administered the needles. (Being on the acupuncture Committee of the National Institutes of Health and vice president of the American Society of Chinese Medicine and The Acupuncture Research Institute, Dr. Chen is quite an acupuncture authority in America.) Four needles were inserted into the subject — two in Hoku and two in Litin, (in between the 2nd and 3rd toes). The first two needles were inserted about one-half inch deep and connected to an acupuncture stimulator; the last two were about one-quarter of an inch deep and being manipulated by hand. The stimulator was a nine-volt batteried electronic pulse generator, set in the frequency of about 3 cycles per second. There was muscular contraction of the hand caused by the electric current. After about twenty minutes, the operation began.

Everything went smoothly during the operation as expected. After the operation the patient said that the operation did not hurt, but she did feel some discomfort. However, there was no nausea, vomiting or hangover. The patient left the hospital after 48 hours.

A CALL FOR MORE BIO-MEDICAL ENGINEERING

In the sphere of Western medicine, we must admit that in the past three hundred years, it has been in great success in its scientific development. This mainly depends on our fantastic achievements of modern engineering techniques. The science synthesizing the fields of biology and engineering is called bio-medical engineering. The term implies that kind of scientific discipline which aims at the understanding of the operation of living systems which are dictated by the needs of human beings or of human society. Although its main role is to develop diagnostic equipment, therapeutic devices, life support systems, etc., its function is to understand rather than to create: to lay the foundation of comprehension on which others can build.* With this foundation of mutual understanding, it can then be incorporated to service, especially in medicine.

Chinese medicine has several thousand years of experience. In its use and application, it is not only simple and economical, but is particularly effective for a certain class of diseases. This is an empirical science, although there are so many unclear questions. Since our ultimate goal is for the benefit of humanity, our foundation should extend to any kind of medicine which can contribute to the enrichment of medical science. Therefore, it is hoped that the science of bio-medical engineering will also be applied to Chinese medicine and be able to unveil its mystery on a solid scientific ground.

Harold Wayland, "Biological Engineering Science and The Three-fold Way" Bio-engineering—An Engineering View, San Francisco Press, Inc., 1968.

REFERENCES (Selected)

BOOKS

Acupuncture Anesthesia, Foreign Language Press, Peking, 1972.

Acupuncture Study Group, Chinese Medical College, *Acupuncture,* The Academy Press Co., Hong Kong, 1970, (in the Chinese language)

Atlas of Human Anatomy, Barnes and Noble, Inc. New York, 1968.

Chan, P., *Acupuncture, Electro-acupuncture, Anesthesia,* 1972.

Chen, C. Y., *History of Chinese Medical Science,* Chinese Medical Institute, Hong Kong, 1968.

Chu Lien, *Modern Acupuncture,* People's Health Publishers, China, 1954, (in the Chinese language).

Fung Tien-yao, *Electro-acupuncture,* The Commercial Press Ltd., Hong Kong, 1967, (in the Chinese language).

Geddes, L. A. and Baker, L. E. *Principles of Applied Biomedical Instrumentation,* John Wiley and Sons, Inc., New York, London, Sydney, 1968.

Hashimoto, M., edited and annotated by Philip Chanellor, *Japanese Acupuncture,* Thorsons Publishers Ltd., 1966.

Ho Shan-mao, *A New Chinese-English Health Medical Dictionary,* Five Continents Publishers Ltd., Taiwan, 1970.

Horn, Joshua S., *Away With All Pests,* Monthly Review Press, 1971.

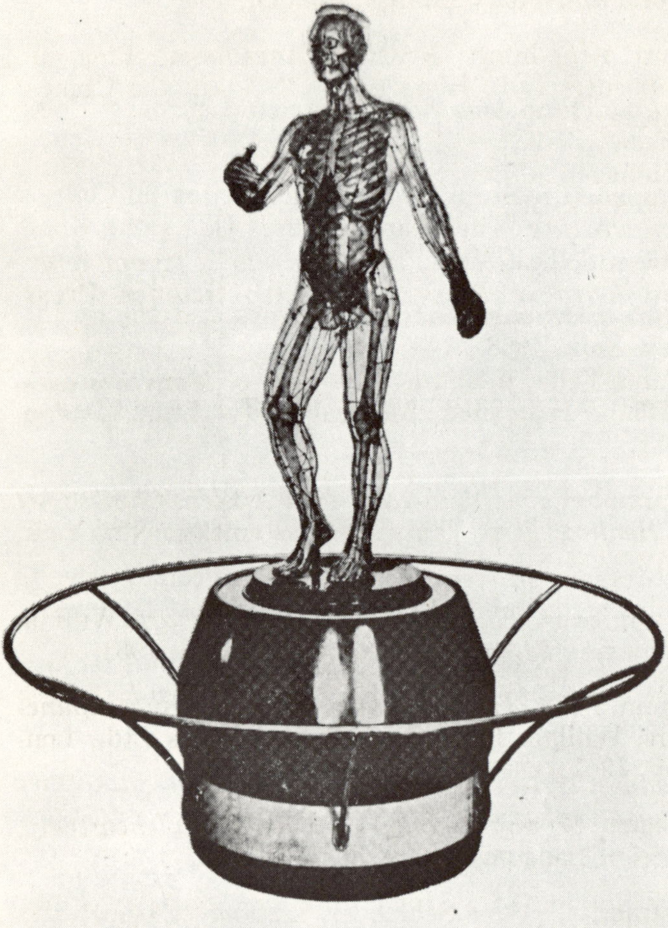

圖 14　經絡、經穴玻璃人。

Huard Pierre and Wong Ming, *Chinese Medicine,* World University Library, London, 1968.

Lam King-hung, *Needling Anesthesia,* Ping Jin Publishers Ltd., Hong Kong, 1971, (in the Chinese language).

Lehninger, Albert L., *Bioenergetics,* W. A. Benjamin, New York, 1965.

Lawsen-Wood, *The Five Elements of Acupuncture and Chinese Massage,* Health Science Press, Rustington, 1966.

Mann, Felix, *Acupuncture—Cure of Many Diseases,* William Heimeman Medical Books Ltd., London, 1971.

Mann, Felix, *Acupuncture—The Ancient Chinese Art of Healing,* First Vantage Books edition, New York, 1972.

Mann, Felix, *The Meridians of Acupuncture,* William Heineman Medical Books Ltd., London, 1964.

Mann, Felix, *The Treatment of Disease By Acupuncture,* William Heineman Medical Books Ltd., London, 1967.

Medical Workers Serving the People Wholeheartedly, Foreign Language Press, Peking, 1971.

Ostrander, S. and Schroeder, L., *Psychic Discoveries Behind the Iron Curtain,* Bantam Books, New York, 1971.

Snow, Edgar, *Red China Today,* Vantage Books, New York, 1971.

Strong, Peter, *Biophysical Measurements,* Tektronix, Inc., Beaverton, Oregon, 1970.

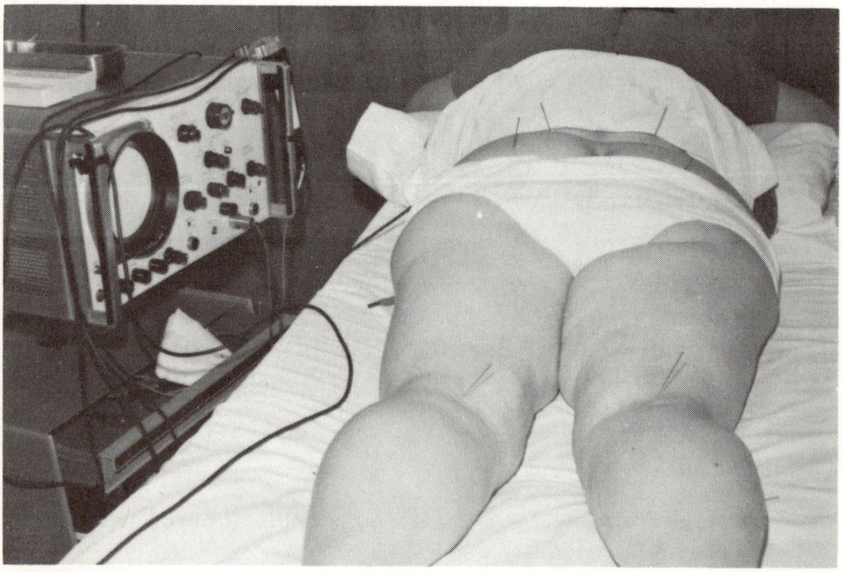

The New Illustrated Medical and Health Encyclopedia, edited by Fishbein, Morris, H. S. Stuttman Co., Inc., New York, 1970.

Wallnofer, H. and Bottauscher, A. V., *Chinese Folk Medicine,* translated by Marion Palmedo, Bell Publishing Co., Inc., New York.

Wu-Wei-ping, *Acupuncture Therapy,* New Asia's Publishing Co., Taipei, 1968.

ADDED REFERENCES

Report From Red China, The New York Times, Avon Books, New York, 1971.

Medicine and Public Health in the People's Republic of China, U. S. Dept. of Health, Education and Welfare, Public Health Service, National Institute of Health, 1972.

All About Acupuncture, Newsweek, August 14, 1972.

The Yellow Emperor's Classic of Internal Medicine, Ilza Veith, The Williams and Wilkins Co., Baltimore, 1949.

The NIH Record, August 1, 1972.

Pain Mechanisms: A New Theory, Malzak and Wall, Science 150, 1965.

Editorial on Acupuncture Anesthesia: Neurogenic Interference Theory, H. C. Tien, World Journal of Psychosynthesis, Vol. 4, No. 4, April 1972.

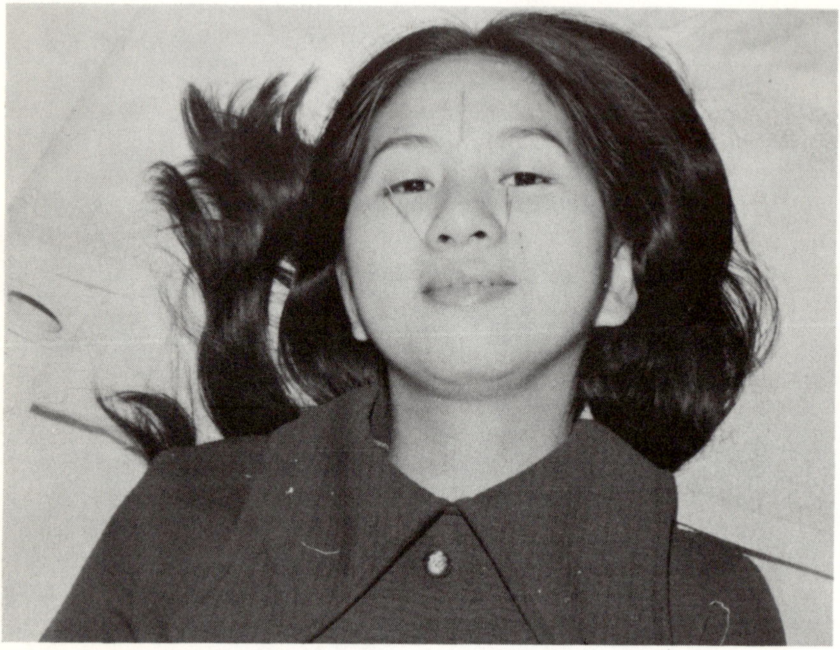

PAPERS

Dimond, E. Grey, *Acupuncture Anesthesia,* Jama, Dec. 6, 1971.

Dimond, E. Grey, *Medical Education and Care in People's Republic of China,* Jama, Dec. 6, 1971.

Fields, Albert, *Acupuncture,* The Lynx Eye, March 1972.

Han, Suyin, *Acupuncture — the Scientific Evidence,* Eastern Horizon, April 1964, Hong Kong.

Shanghai Acupunctural Anesthesia Co-ordinating Group, *Acupuncture Anesthesia,* Red Flag, Vol. 9, 1971. (in Chinese)

People's Liberation Army Hospital, *Acupuncture Anesthesia,* Red Flag, Vol. 9, 1971. (in Chinese)

People's Liberation Army Hospital, *Acupuncture Anesthesia,* Canton Headquarter, Vol. 9, 1971. (in Chinese)

Research Institute of Acupuncture and Moxibustion, *Chinese Medical Theory and the Method of Treatment by Acupuncture and Moxibustion,* Academy of Traditional Chinese Medicine, Peking.

Mann, Felix, "Chinese Traditional Medicine, A Practitioner's View", *The China Quarterly,* July-September, 1965, London.

Kwan, C., "On Acupuncture Anesthesia", *Ming Pao Monthly,* Nov. 1971, Hong Kong. (in Chinese)

Topping, Audrey, "Acupuncture", *Vogue,* Jan. 1, 1972.

Peking Acupunctural Anesthesia Co-ordinating Group, "The Principle of Acupunctural Anesthesia, *Peking Review*, February 25, 1972, Peking.

Research Institute of Acupuncture and Moxibustion Academy of Traditional Chinese Medicine, *The Efficacy of Acupuncture and Moxibustion*, Peking.

Yao, H.H., "The Secret of Acupuncture", *Ming Pao Monthly*, Sept. 1971, Hong Kong. (in Chinese)

STATEMENT OF RESPONSIBILITY BY AUTHOR AND PUBLISHER

This book is merely a discussion of acupuncture and some of its ramifications. Since acupuncture is considered in the experimental stage in the United States, the Author and the Publisher will not assume responsibility and/or liability for acupuncture use in any way by anyone.